Employed Physician Networks

Employed Physician Networks

A Guide to Building Strategic Advantage, Value, and Financial Sustainability

David W. Miller
Terrence R. McWilliams
Travis C. Ansel

ACHE Management Series

Acquisitions editor: Janet Davis; Manuscript editor: Jane Calayag; Project manager: Michael Noren; Cover designer: Brad Norr; Layout: Cepheus Edmondson

Found an error or a typo? We want to know! Please email it to hapbooks@ache.org, mentioning the book's title and putting "Book Error" in the subject line.

For photocopying and copyright information, please contact Copyright Clearance Center at www.copyright.com or at (978) 750-8400.

Health Administration Press
A division of the Foundation of the American
    College of Healthcare Executives
300 S. Riverside Plaza, Suite 1900
Chicago, IL 60606–6698
(312) 424-2800

Contents

Acknowledgments

SEVERAL INDIVIDUALS HAVE contributed greatly to the development of this book. John Hill and Neal Barker, each a partner at HSG, and Davis Creech, director, have contributed many thoughts through their work with the firm's clients. Their ideas are particularly prevalent as we discuss the eight elements of successful groups and the assessment of employed networks.

Thanks to the HSG staff, who contributed ideas and helped the firm stay on track while we were writing. Thanks are due in particular to Sarah Brunton, whose efforts to edit and organize were invaluable. Thanks also to Donna Russell, who edited the book for us.

Thanks to Janet Davis and the editors at Health Administration Press for their direction and support. Thanks also to Carson Dye, who coached us on working with HAP and got us off to a great start.

A special thanks to our client executives who allowed us to identify their organization in case studies and other references: Chris Candio and Scott Johnson at St. Luke's Hospital; Bill Griffin at Halifax Health; William Melahn, MD, at St. Claire Regional; Lynn Miller at Geisinger Health; Chris Roederer at Tampa General Hospital; Jeff Samz at Huntsville Health; and Neil Thornbury at TJ Samson Community Hospital. Additional thanks to those clients who contributed to our thinking and insights, even if we did not use them in a case study.

Last but not least, thanks to our wives, who put up with a lot of writing during really odd hours: Karen Miller, Lisa McWilliams, and Lindsey Ansel.

PART I

The Basics

THIS SECTION INCLUDES chapters 1 through 4, which present the fundamental concepts for building employed physician networks. Specifically, these chapters discuss the following:

- Factors that have brought hospitals and health systems to the point at which employed networks are a critical challenge
- Six phases of employed network evolution, from novice to high performing
- Key barriers to progressing to the next level of performance
- Eight elements of successful employed networks

All of these concepts play an important role in making your network a strategic asset for your organization.

CHAPTER 1

Introduction

In the middle of difficulty lies opportunity.

—Albert Einstein

OVER THE PAST decade, market forces have pushed both health-care organizations (hospitals and health systems) and physicians to aggressively pursue employment. This book focuses on how to make physician employment a success, discussing, among other things, how to get a return on your investment, how to build a strategic asset so that you can confidently prepare for the future, and how to create a high-performing physician group in partnership with your physicians.

The concept of physician partnership is crucial to a healthcare organization's success. Without engaged physicians or a systematic approach to tapping into their knowledge and growing their capabilities, the organization may not be successful (or operational) for long. The evolving market and governmental requirements, with an increasing focus on value-based care, guarantee that organizations will need to engage physicians in a different way. This book will help you define that way.

GROWTH OF PHYSICIAN EMPLOYMENT

In 2016, more than half of all physicians were employed by an entity such as a hospital. According to the American Medical Association,

2016 was the first year in which fewer than half of all practicing physicians in the United States owned their medical practice, with only 47.1 percent reporting ownership (Kane 2017). Four major factors are behind that trend.

First, the complexity of operating in today's marketplace is driving physicians into the arms of large organizations. Constantly changing quality data requirements, electronic health record requirements, and insurer burdens have created a market where small, stand-alone practices are no longer positioned for success. The only exceptions are lucrative specialties, such as urology or gastroenterology, with ownership of ancillary services.

Second, private practices must consider the revenue challenges of independence. If the practice is small, it is likely to be treated unfairly or taken advantage of by insurers during rate negotiations. Joining a larger organization with more negotiating power improves the practice's financial performance immediately.

Third, newly minted physicians, who are often in debt, have certain expectations. Setting up a private practice after completing residency is daunting, unless a lucrative specialty practice expresses an interest in partnering. The security of hospital employment can be a magnet. The pull is further reinforced by the fact that a healthcare organization is likely to value a new physician much more than a private practice could.

Fourth, healthcare organizations have strategic and service needs. In most markets, depending on private practices to fill these needs is unrealistic; physician employment is necessary to preserve the organization and serve its community. Even in markets where private practices have traditionally thrived, a market or competitive factor eventually challenges the viability of the practice's cooperative arrangement with the hospital or health system. Most organizations need to employ physicians if they wish to remain in the healthcare delivery business.

Healthcare organizations employ physicians as a strategy for a broad range of issues, including the following:

1. To strengthen the competitive position in a service line or a geographic region
2. To improve or preserve patient access to services, thereby helping to control patient flow (To this end, the organization may engage in new provider recruitment, employment of incumbent physicians to solidify their private practice, or succession planning.)
3. To fill a service needed by the community, even when the organization derives no business advantage from it
4. To add a new capability or to upgrade the quality of the care in a specialty (See Miller and Johnston [2018] for a case study of Huntsville Health and its efforts to achieve board understanding and acceptance of its physician employment strategy.)

Given that physician employment has become more prevalent, this book's focus on building a strong physician group and integrating that group into the organization's overall business model is timely.

PATIENT PERSPECTIVE

By better integrating care, employed physician networks provide a great vehicle for improving quality of care. For most healthcare executives, these networks offer an opportunity to make a significant contribution to patient care during their career. Inevitably, the old private practice model created inappropriate variation in quality and uncoordinated care. This is not to say that physicians were not doing what they thought was right; rather, aside from a loosely organized medical staff, no established chassis or framework was in place that drove them to look for better practices. At their best, employed networks are that chassis.

Integrated employed networks can improve access to care, although organizational bureaucracies and poor management infrastructure can make this objective elusive. With organizational capital enabling their development, networks are given opportunities to expand access. Employed networks are better able than most private practices to obtain the physician/provider resources that patients need, whether that care is in a physician's office, an emergency department, or a hospital unit for a consultation. Under this system, many patients can access care in their communities that would not be available if the market were solely driven by private practice.

In addition, because physicians are linked culturally and electronically, they can better coordinate patient care among primary care physicians and specialists. Making referrals becomes easier, and a group willing to define member expectations related to speed of appointments can improve it further. The ability to move patients to less busy providers is another opportunity to improve access. However, access is not a given. Bureaucracy combined with underinvestment in management infrastructure often gets in the way of smooth patient care. A management dyad working together with engaged physicians can help overcome this challenge. The implications for greater throughput are obviously attractive to executive leaders as well.

Surprisingly, delivering consistent, high-quality patient experiences is the most elusive objective for many physician networks. Because of financial and quality challenges, patient experience often gets deprioritized; it is simply not perceived to be so bad that action is required. But the promise of excellent patient experience remains high, as employed networks build one registration system and one electronic record with a patient portal, while also promoting consistent patient interactions. Excellent patient experience is a key to a strong, valued brand for a network.

STRATEGIC PERSPECTIVE

The primary reason that employed networks are important to healthcare organizations is their strategic value. One of our hospital CEO clients defined his objective as creating a "strategic weapon."

Organizations use these groups in a variety of strategic ways. First, they use the groups to generate volume. We list volume first because it is the original motivation of most healthcare executives. A physician may have become employed when she was thinking about retiring or leaving town, or when she was unable to sustain the practice, or when the hospital needed to expand a service line. All of these motivations are tied to volume.

The second way organizations use these groups is to improve quality. Organizations that have moved beyond the initial network evolutionary phases have discovered that an integrated, multispecialty group can address complex quality issues in a way that small private practices cannot.

The third way that organizations use groups—and this is the Holy Grail in today's world—is to manage risk. We can define a high-performing group in terms of its capability to deliver predictable quality and costs. This capability opens the door to a different financial model, where physicians and their hospitals can thrive economically by managing care.

The employed network can also open the door to a new focus on community health. The ability to work with employers and defined populations to improve health creates a new model for care. We do not have all the answers for building that model, but we do believe that, through an employed network, an organization can work with physicians and other providers to create a model for the community. It just needs the right forum. Employed networks are a great forum to deal with this challenge.

Some people believe that clinically integrated networks (CINs) can realize that promise. With the right players, they may. But divergent incentives and varying cultures within CINs make doing so more difficult. CINs may be required in some markets because of the mix of employed physicians and private-practice physicians. But all things being equal, fully integrated groups have a better chance of performing well.

FINANCIAL PERSPECTIVE

In the early stages of employing physicians, many healthcare organizations focus on finances. Losing large amounts of money will do that! Focusing on long-term strategy is difficult when financial losses are bringing about challenges and disrupting board relationships.

Many types of errors drive financial losses in novice groups, but most can be chalked up to lack of investment in management infrastructure. That can mean not hiring the right numbers and types of people or treating the revenue cycle as an extension of the organization's main operation. Poorly conceived compensation plans can also drive losses, as can declines in physician productivity.

Many organizations, especially those performing well financially, have reconciled themselves to these losses, viewing them as a cost of doing business. Others are slowly gaining insights into the losses and managing the root causes. Some are moving to the next stage of employment by experimenting with one-sided risk to achieve some upside, whereas others are engaging physicians for their insights on financial sustainability.

PHYSICIAN PERSPECTIVE

The ability to tap and gain insights from physicians and other providers is a core competency that organizations must develop if they are to wring maximum value from employed networks. It is central to a network's long-term success.

Cultural barriers exist from both the employed physician side and the healthcare executive side. On the physician side, some physicians want to sell their practice because they are sick of dealing with management issues. One of the reasons you employed them is to gain their insights into strategy, operations, and quality, so don't let them abdicate their management and leadership roles! It never goes well. On the executive side, many executives are wary of physicians and have adopted the mentality of not wanting the "inmates to run the prison." Fostering this mind-set prohibits you from developing a high-performing network. It means you and the leadership team are restraining the group's ability to achieve success and limiting its strategic value.

Physician engagement is important for another reason: It fosters physicians' sense of well-being and control and thus promotes provider retention. In employed networks where physician engagement is high and built on a common purpose and supportive culture, retention is more likely. Building a supportive culture while still holding physicians accountable is one of the biggest challenges physician executives face. More on that later.

Changing incentives in the US healthcare system are making physician engagement a necessity. The need to work with physicians to manage care quality and related financial incentives will continue to drive the need for greater integration.

HOW TO USE THIS BOOK

Our goal for this book is to serve as a primary resource on this topic. You may read it cover to cover, but you may also use it as a reference and read only the chapters most relevant to your situation. For example, in part II, the six phases of network evolution are discussed. (Chapter 2 begins our exploration of this evolution.) If you are at the third phase, Operational Chaos, you may skip to chapter 7 and skim the chapters on the earlier phases. Throughout the six phases, management expertise, level of physician engagement, and core capabilities will change and grow. The tactics to consider and the dashboard metrics to track will also evolve. Use the book to focus predominantly on where you are going, not where you have been.

At the end of most chapters, cases and/or additional resources are included. These bonus materials allow a deeper dive into particular issues.

Most hospitals want practical advice and useful guidance, rather than a prescription. This book will help you define a plan for your group—a plan that fits the unique culture of your organization and the accountabilities of each member of your group's leadership team. The sample dashboards (see chapter 12) as well as our recommendations on areas of focus, depending on where you are in your evolution, should aid the leadership team and other executives. Many healthcare executives have limited experience with physician groups. They may have years of experience with hospital issues but be relatively unprepared to shape a physician group. We hope to accelerate not only their progress but also their confidence in this endeavor.

For health system leaders dealing with multiple physician groups spread over a wide geography, the book offers a common framework and language for managing those groups. Our growth curve model (see chapter 2) recognizes that subsets of a group may be at different points in their evolution and that variation in performance exists, but it still guides leaders in defining a common ultimate destination.

Central to your success is a shared vision of what you want the group to be (see chapter 4). Our suggested time frame for vision discussions is ten years. Some will disagree with that time frame, believing that projecting a decade into the future is impossible. We acknowledge that such a projection will require some changes, but we reject that it is impossible. Many elements of the future market are predictable. In ten years, your group will have to do a better job at coordinating care. It will need more robust data. It will need to manage outcomes and costs more effectively. It will need to learn to manage risk. Capturing the insights of physicians about how to address these challenges will be essential, and accountability must increase.

Ultimately, we hope to help organizations improve patient care by

- organizing and guiding their employed networks,
- supporting physicians in how they work and where they focus, and
- recognizing that great patient care must begin with physician engagement and physician well-being.

We expect this book to provide a route to a successful collaboration between physicians and the healthcare organization.

CONCLUSION

This book represents our best take on where employed groups are today and where they may be tomorrow. At our consulting practice, HSG, our perspective has been informed through extensive experience working with hospitals and health systems that have built a network. We have learned and continue to learn a lot from our clients, and we gain new insights every time we visit these groups. We hope you will share with us your thoughts and experiences about your own journey. We also welcome your feedback about this book, particularly the insights you think we missed.

REFERENCES

Kane, C. 2017. "Updated Data on Physician Practice Arrangements: Physician Ownership Drops Below 50 Percent." Policy Research Perspectives. Accessed January 2018. www.ama-assn.org/sites/default/files/media-browser/public/health-policy/PRP-2016-physician-benchmark-survey.pdf.

Miller, D., and L. Johnston. 2018. "Does Your Board Understand Why Physicians Are Employed?" *Becker's Hospital Review.* Published February 22. www.beckershospitalreview.com/hospital-management-administration/does-your-board-understand-why-physicians-are-employed.html.

CHAPTER 2

Evolution of Employed Networks

We are the facilitators of our own creative evolution.

—Bill Hicks

EMPLOYED PHYSICIAN NETWORKS evolve over time, in response to market and healthcare organization requirements. From working with hundreds of groups, we have learned that this evolution follows a somewhat predictable pattern. The benefit of that insight is significant: If you understand the pattern, you can accelerate through the phases of evolution that will inevitably occur. Predictable issues will emerge that you should tackle according to an assessment of your group's current state. This chapter provides an overview of the evolutionary phases; chapters 5 through 10 will discuss the six phases in detail.

This chapter introduces the growth curve model, which provides a method for assessing your network's evolution and determining its current phase of development. Because employed physician networks are a relatively new endeavor for many healthcare organizations, having a common framework for understanding the endeavor's progress is of value. This model can drive performance toward goals, articulate to physicians their place in the system, and define the priorities for investments. For health systems with multiple networks, the model establishes a common language throughout, while acknowledging variations in performance and progress.

With the knowledge afforded by the model, the network can not only create a plan but also prioritize its activities for moving to the next phase or the next level.

THE GROWTH CURVE MODEL

Exhibit 2.1 identifies the six phases through which employed networks progress. The x-axis addresses time, with groups generally progressing over time from the Novice phase (left of the exhibit) to the High-Performing phase (right). Networks could certainly regress, but that is seldom seen in the market.

The y-axis generally represents the number of employed networks in each phase. Although the graph is depicted as a bell curve, the

Exhibit 2.1: Six Phases of Employed Network Evolution

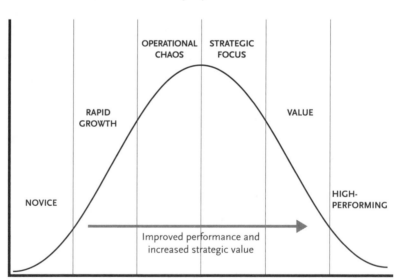

distribution of the phases is slightly different in reality. The largest cohort is in the third phase, Operational Chaos. According to self-reports, executives most often consider themselves in that phase, though they are also reporting greater strategic progress. In reality, many networks exhibit characteristics that span multiple phases. Some aspects of their performance may mirror Operational Chaos, but they may also be focusing on strategic challenges, a hallmark of the fourth phase.

Novice Phase

This phase describes new groups. Management is not strong, and physicians do not act as a group. The healthcare organization may be dabbling in physician employment, forced to do it as a reaction to market realities. These groups are, in reality, individual practices with a common tax ID number. Most organizations have moved beyond this phase.

Rapid Growth Phase

In this second phase, the organization is aggressively growing physician employment. The focus is short term. Management is making deals and ensuring the organization does not run afoul of regulatory requirements. Strategic employment is likely pursued because it will build a service line or add volume. An overarching plan of how or where the group should grow is rare. Developing systems that will help the group operate successfully is given minimal importance. The person charged with "running" the network likely is a department head or, worse, an executive who is already juggling multiple responsibilities. This loose or underdeveloped management infrastructure is the precursor to the third phase.

Operational Chaos Phase

At this phase, network growth has outstripped management capabilities. The corollary is that the organization is increasingly struggling with subsidies, many of which are unexpected. That likely reality is creating tension at the board level as well. Healthcare executives are likely to react in one of three ways.

First, they may acknowledge that the resources committed to managing the group are inadequate. Executives often struggle to fix this, as they do not know where to find good practice managers or how to screen them. The capabilities required to manage a network are not the same as those required to manage a hospital.

Second, they may slow down physician employment. In the face of board concerns and pressure, halting or slowing down the network's growth until a plan is in place may be prudent to mitigate financial concerns. However, this reaction can lead to long-term strategic mistakes, especially when competitors do not share the same concerns.

Third, they may cut the network's costs. However, office staffing that is too lean can hurt throughput, and often these cost-containment measures decrease revenue (or potential revenue) more than they reduce expenses. Staffing that is too lean can also be detrimental to staff and provider retention.

Strategic Focus Phase

The management infrastructure is now maturing to meet the requirements of the network. At this point, physician leaders may be in dyad relationships with practice managers, although that sometimes does not happen until the Value phase.

In this phase, networks start working on strategic challenges and engaging physicians and physician leaders in those discussions. Many groups begin to discuss their long-term vision or their need to evolve over five to ten years. They also address strategic issues related to group growth and expansion. Ideally, this phase is when the groundwork is set in place for quality improvement and population health.

Two issues tend to arise in the Strategic Focus phase. The first is the culling of physicians who may not be able to deliver on expectations in the long term. This action is a response to a challenge created in the Rapid Growth phase, when some hospitals employ any physician with patients to admit. The second is establishing a working relationship between the network and private physicians (a significant challenge explored in chapter 11).

Value Phase

In this phase, the physicians are fully engaged, and the network is well integrated and learning how to produce value. A big part of the discussion is selecting what care model (e.g., team-based care or medical home) to adopt that will produce value and reaching consensus on how to provide that care. This is the beginning of risk taking, which many groups have attempted prematurely, with disastrous results. In this phase, networks also enhance their ability to deliver consistent experiences.

The quality improvement and patient experience capabilities of the network are more robust. More complex care management and care coordination challenges are effectively addressed. Such progress allows the healthcare organization to better integrate the network with its managed care strategy, even making employed physicians and private practice allies central to that strategy.

High-Performing Phase

A High-Performing network can reliably manage outcomes and costs. It has a strong, consistent culture that drives its success. Its vision is clear. Its operations range from stable to strong. Great patient experiences make it a provider of choice. And it is capable of managing risk.

Inevitable Learning Curve

On rare occasion, a healthcare organization may avoid the learning curve of network building if it has the benefit of an especially insightful network leader. Such a leader may be a physician with a clear vision of what the network needs to be, or an experienced practice manager who recognizes the infrastructure needed.

In most cases, however, the learning curve is inevitable, and it could be steep under the following conditions:

- *The leader is unable to exert influence.* Influence may be acquired by earning the trust of the organizational CEO and having a successful record of accomplishment. Being knowledgeable about employed networks is not enough. The leader must show that knowledge is applied and the advice from experts is heeded.
- *The organization lacks a coherent physician culture.* Even if the medical staff has a culture, it rarely (if ever) mimics the culture of a fully integrated network. Developing a cohesive culture is never an overnight task, and its absence stunts network progress.
- *The leader lacks management expertise.* Organizational leaders don't know what they don't know. Many have confidence in their own ability, but in reality they may have no reason to be confident in the employed network arena.

WHERE IS YOUR NETWORK ON THE GROWTH CURVE?

Most executives, when faced with the growth curve model, instinctively estimate where their efforts fall on the curve. The language itself, and HSG's description of what executives experience at each phase, provides a general direction.

Consider the following general questions as you evaluate your network's progress along the growth curve. Go beyond your basic gut feel during your assessment.

1. Do you anticipate significant growth? Will the group ultimately be much larger?
2. What is your assessment of the size, depth, and capabilities of the management team?
   - Do you have the management team that can lead the day-to-day operations?
   - Do you have the dyads that can lead you to high performance?
3. Is financial performance under control?
   - Do you understand your performance compared with benchmarks?
   - Do you understand the strategic value of physician subsidies?
   - Do productivity and compensation correlate?
   - Is the revenue cycle under control?
4. Does the network retain referrals when appropriate?
   - Do physician leaders understand referral patterns?
   - Are they working with their peers to retain referrals when appropriate?
   - Do you have the mind-set needed to earn referrals?
5. Are your practices connected through a common electronic health record (EHR)?
   - Are data from the EHR being leveraged to the benefit of patients and their care?
   - Are you creating the capability to manage to payer metrics?
6. Are physicians involved in leadership?
   - Is there a physician advisory council?
   - Is there a physician executive in direct line management of the group?
   - Are network physicians involved with the hospital or health system leadership?
7. Is there a common vision among physicians and executives about what the group must become?
   - Do physicians and nonphysician executives have the same expectations?

- Have physicians helped create those expectations?
8. Is the employed physician network tackling value-based care challenges for the group and the organization?
   - Is the network incorporating them into its vision and annual plan?
   - Does your compensation system reward these efforts and results?
9. In its dashboard, does the network address performance on cost and quality?
   - Are those measures progressing over time so that the network is focused on issues important to patients and payers?
   - Over time, have you seen an accelerating sophistication in the dashboard?

HSG uses three assessment approaches—data reviews, interviews, and surveys—to gauge where a network falls on the curve and to prioritize improvement plans. These tools help identify the capabilities of the group, tracking its progress to the right side of the curve.

Data Reviews

Productivity and throughput can easily be assessed by looking at network data. The ease with which management can produce these data tells us a lot about the network infrastructure and capabilities.

Interviews

Some topics are so complex that interviews with subject matter experts are necessary to gain insights. For example, multiple issues could drive poor revenue cycle performance. The complexity of that process—from intake in the physician office to working claims denials and posting of final payments—makes determining the issues impossible without detailed discussions with the relevant players. A deep dive into the data accompanied by interviews with the functional leaders can be very useful.

Surveys

Surveys are completed by a broad range of constituents and provide further insights as well. We use two levels of surveys:

1. Network Evaluation Survey (appendix) provides a broad overview of the network and is aimed at executives responsible for its operations and results, as well as physician leaders. Differences in perceptions are often identified and offer useful information.
2. Practice Operations Survey is geared toward practice managers and individual practices. It explores business systems and capabilities.

Links to the Network Evaluation Survey and the Practice Operations Survey are included in the Additional Resources section at the end of the chapter.

CONCLUSION

Understanding how networks evolve and where your network falls along the growth curve will help your organization anticipate and prepare for what's ahead. It will also facilitate efforts to engage physicians in current and future initiatives because it shows them how they fit into the organization and how they can contribute to its success. Involved physicians feel some level of control in an increasingly complex healthcare marketplace.

ADDITIONAL RESOURCES

Assessment Tools

Network Evaluation Survey: http://hsgadvisors.com/Network
  EvaluationSurvey.

Practice Operations Survey: http://hsgadvisors.com/PracticeOperations
  Survey.

Webinar with Halifax Health

"Building High-Performing Networks": http://info.hsgadvisors.com/
  high-performing-network-webinar.

White Paper

HSG. 2017. "Physician Growth Phases—Accelerating the Performance
  of Your Network." http://hsgadvisors.com/thought-leadership/
  white-paper/physician-network-growth-phases/.

CASES

The following cases illustrate the concepts discussed in the
chapter. The healthcare organizations featured in this section
have had a long-term relationship with our consulting practice,
HSG, and have given us permission to discuss their employed
physician network journey.

Halifax Health

Halifax Health, a two-hospital public system based in Day-
tona Beach, Florida, had a growing but unorganized employed
physician network. The network employed more than 120 providers on the 740-member medical staff. Working with HSG,
Halifax systematically attacked its problem areas, stabilized

operations, and then turned its focus to the employed network's strategy in the marketplace.

Despite a growing commitment to physician employment, Halifax had no centralized management infrastructure for the group. Management of physicians was within service lines, which led to inconsistent clinical standards, performance expectations, and physician engagement. Physicians were disengaged from operations and had limited input into organizational or network strategy.

The network's revenue cycle was integrated into the hospital revenue cycle and disconnected from practice operations. Not unexpectedly, performance suffered. Using metrics was impossible as the data from various billing systems were inconsistent or nonexistent.

Approach

With HSG's guidance, the network team first built a robust management infrastructure, adding an executive director and a financial analyst to accelerate its understanding of the financial challenges. The network's leadership core worked with hospital executives to shift incumbent physician staff into the "right seat." Next, it enhanced communications both among the practices and between practices and executives. Facilitating this effort were the dashboards and management reports the team developed. Data development was not a quick process, as financial statements were not produced on a timely basis, but the availability of current data and information vastly improved the team's ability to manage the practices.

The rest of the approach consisted of creating policies and procedures, providing a copious amount of staff training, and strengthening payer credentialing to support the improvement of the revenue cycle.

continued

After one year, physician engagement took on a greater focus. The network assembled a Physician Advisory Council to provide input. Starting with the creation of a charter and mission, the group moved on to planning the creation of a unified electronic medical record (EMR), standardizing operations, marketing the group, and establishing quality indicators and incentives related to the Merit-Based Incentive Payment System.

Working with the physicians and key executives, the team developed a three-year strategic plan. A core component of the plan was to bolster primary care services, as the network's early growth had a specialty focus designed to support hospital service lines.

Results and Impact

The most significant outcome is that Halifax leaders now believe, correctly, that the network is stable and its leadership is being developed. Executives have a better understanding of the operations, performance, and strategic potential of the group.

Many tangible results were achieved, including the following:

- Network losses have declined by 8 percent, although the transition to a single EMR may challenge that.
- Productivity increased by 2 percent in 2017, as a result of managing expectations and gaining greater control over scheduling.
- The network's primary care base grew with the addition of six new practices.
- Management now receives timely data on practice operations.

Working with the physicians, Halifax is currently targeting further operational improvements and creating a clear vision of the network's role within the organization.

Geisinger Health System

In 2015, HSG conducted a productivity assessment on more than 30 clinical departments, evaluating physician and all-provider productivity and office staffing ratios against AMGA and Medical Group Management Association benchmarks. Geisinger Health System, headquartered in Danville, Pennsylvania, targeted physician productivity to exceed the 65th percentile and deemed office staffing ratios between the 50th and 75th percentiles as acceptable. When the analyses of all clinical departments were completed, we summarized the data and ranked the individual departments according to all-provider productivity. The productivity ranking produced an interesting insight regarding associated staffing ratios. For all but one department that achieved an all-provider productivity ranking above the 70th percentile, the clinical support staffing ratios compared with external benchmarks indicated that the offices were overstaffed. The one exception was the psychiatry department.

The individual department interview and data-review process revealed that these highly productive departments used their support staff to their maximum capabilities, and the departments attributed their success to the level of staffing they were afforded. This finding uniformly applied to all of the highly productive areas. The bottom-line lessons from this assessment were (1) that great care should be exercised when interpreting only one facet of office function and making decisions on the basis of that one facet and (2) that excess staff relative to benchmarks may not actually be excess and in fact may be the reason the office is able to perform well on patient throughput. In Geisinger's case, evaluation based on the staffing ratio might have led to efforts to decrease the number of clinical support staff to be in line with external benchmarks, but this could have been detrimental to clinical functions and outcomes.

CHAPTER 3

Barriers to
High Performance

A bruise is a lesson ... and each lesson makes us better.

—George R. R. Martin

ADVANCING AN EMPLOYED network toward the High-Performing
phase of the growth curve model (introduced in chapter 2) is not a
simple process. High-performing physician groups are rare. Biases
in favor of private practice, regulations discouraging the corporate
practice of medicine, and economic challenges of physician employment all contribute to making employed networks a resource few
healthcare organizations have succeeded in building.

Barriers abound. In this chapter, we discuss these barriers, highlighting
two that seem to be almost universal: lack of management infrastructure
and lack of a shared vision. Although less common, a third major barrier—the lack of strong physician leadership—can impede a network's
evolution from the Novice phase to the High-Performing phase. We also
examine six tactical and implementation issues that can slow progress.

LACK OF MANAGEMENT INFRASTRUCTURE

As networks grow and advance to the Operational Chaos phase,
lack of management infrastructure can become an enormous barrier.

Management issues are often a direct result of the way the network was built. Rather than forming a network as a strategic initiative, healthcare organizations are more likely to establish one as a defensive strategy to prevent the loss of practitioners to competitors or other communities. In such instances, not much thought is devoted to how the group should be managed over the long run. This kind of oversight sets the stage for four major management deficiencies:

1. *Manager shortage.* Most networks have fewer managers and supervisors than the benchmarks suggest. The Medical Group Management Association multispecialty group standard, for example, calls for one general administrative manager (including a working manager) per 2.7 physicians. After a practice is employed, many healthcare organizations simply keep the preemployment management structure in place; this is the same structure that struggled to address market changes and was partially responsible for the practice pursuing employment in the first place. Reinforcing this weakness is management's ever-present focus on reducing full-time equivalents.

    When organizations do put more managers in place, they tend to select people without physician practice experience. The typical approach is to appoint trusted individuals with demonstrated success in their hospital-based roles and depend on their ability to adapt to practice management, a very different business model. Sometimes the approach works, but often it does not.

2. *Lack of staff capabilities.* Employed networks struggle with this issue from two perspectives. First, the supply of managers with physician practice experience is limited. In almost every community, today's groups are much larger than their historic predecessors, but few executives are available with the breadth of experience required to manage such large networks. Often, only managers with experience in small practices are available. Identifying

which of these administrators can grow to lead big groups is tricky at best.

Second, many struggles stem from the assumption that a good hospital manager can run a physician practice. In reality, the differences between running a hospital and running a practice are significant, particularly with regard to the revenue cycle. Hospital managers are experienced in handling big accounts with the help of well-trained department staff. Typically, the smaller accounts of physician practices require a higher level of attention, and poorly paid front-office staff at private practices often lack the baseline training required to do this job. Thus, the revenue cycle process causes many headaches in the early stages of employed network development.

3. *Lack of accountability for functions.* Under-resourcing and dubious accountability typically result when the network's needs are served from an organizational department. Universally, the network should have dedicated resources for finance and quality. Resources that enable financial analysis and direct control of the revenue cycle are generally good investments with positive returns, and so are quality resources that help measure, monitor, and meet value-based and patient care improvement goals. Localizing these resources in the practices engenders physician ownership as well.

4. *Absence of dyad management.* Dyad management, which is discussed in later chapters, refers to co-leadership by a physician, who's in charge of the clinical aspects, and a manager or administrator, who oversees the business operations. Almost uniformly, early entrants into physician employment discount the importance of engaging physician leaders. Priorities such as acquisition, fair market value estimates, practice staff transition to the organizational payroll, and employee benefits can overwhelm the executive team. Esoteric issues such as

setting up the physician leadership role and initiating its function become distant concerns. Physicians must be part of the network management infrastructure; they must guide the clinical aspect of the venture, while their dyad partners lead the business side. In addition, a broad physician panel needs to be engaged through an advisory council or similar group. Too often, physicians disengage from administration, relieved that the organization has stepped in. This disconnect ultimately leads to significant physician dissatisfaction and suboptimal network performance.

Poor network management causes a lot of chaos within physician practices, and working in a poorly run environment takes a toll. At worst, physicians may leave out of frustration, forcing the group to recruit replacements, who are likely unknown quantities. At best, physicians may become apathetic and disengage from the broader issues where their input is needed.

Management deficiencies also limit the ability to drive and manage change. If network managers are so busy attending meeting after meeting and putting out the fire du jour, they are merely trying not to drive the group into a ditch, so to speak. They have no time for the bigger, strategic picture—how the network must evolve to realize long-term objectives.

Groups that have invested in more managers often fail to include physicians in the management mix. Part of the reason is related to budget: Physicians are expensive resources who need to produce clinical revenue. The other part of the reason involves the inability to identify appropriate physician leaders. Outside of observing who succeeds as a medical staff leader, many executives have limited experience and expertise in evaluating potential physician leaders, assessing their capabilities and temperament, and creating a leadership development plan for multiple physicians.

Another barrier for executives is fear of losing control. Empowering physician leadership has many benefits but also carries some risk. An executive must be secure in her role to empower physicians to help lead the network.

The net result of underinvestment in management talent is subsidies. Under the best of circumstances, network losses can be large. But when a group is poorly managed, losses can become massive. When we at HSG get a call from an executive frantic about losses, we instinctively know the network's management infrastructure is the most likely culprit.

Solving this issue is not simple. The path to a solution involves, first, defining the infrastructure plan. What management positions are needed, based on an assessment of both the numbers and special expertise required? Investing in subject matter experts, financial analytics resources, and quality improvement tools is valuable. Quality resources are especially worthwhile when coordinated with organizational resources and focused on how the practices fit into the continuum of care. Information technology (IT) resources are also crucial investments, ensuring that practice managers have some control over when IT issues get addressed, rather than waiting in a big queue of all the organizational IT problems.

With an infrastructure plan in place, the second step toward a solution is sourcing candidates. Finding people with the right skills is a key concern, given the dearth of available talent. In many cases, hiring a recruiter is a wise investment. Professional recruiters understand the skills and traits required for the job. They ask the right questions and are trained to probe candidates' qualifications to determine their depth of knowledge.

One other infrastructure issue worth discussing is the ambiguous organizational reporting structure. When HSG consultants at physician forums ask doctors whom they report to, we often get blank stares. In many organizations (especially if physicians have been told "nothing will change" with employment), the reporting relationships are left unaddressed. Physicians, however, need to understand how they fit into the organization and to whom they are accountable. Without that accountability, building a multispecialty network that can work with the organization to address market challenges is next to impossible.

LACK OF SHARED VISION

Health system and hospital executives who have not engaged their physicians in discussions about how the network should evolve are allowing the group to remain unfocused or focused solely on finances. In this situation, no commonly accepted plan, long-term vision, or guidelines exist for what executives, physicians, and the board want the network to be.

Typically, executives want to retain patient volume, help physicians who have been loyal, and expand recruitment to private practices (which are drying up in many markets). Physicians want job stability, some level of guaranteed income, and none of the operational and administrative burdens from new regulations. Many board members pine for the days when hospitals did not employ doctors, but they agree to pursue physician employment to meet community needs that would otherwise go unmet, to provide emergency department coverage, and to secure the patient volume needed for financial stability. These players are simply not on the same page.

Without a shared vision, there can be no concerted effort to improve care coordination. Few networks focus on care coordination in the early stages of development, but it is a bedrock of the group's long-term existence. Without a vision, care is delivered the way it has always been delivered, reliant on the best efforts and skills of individual physicians but with no coordination and no system in place for physicians and the organization to learn from each other. Of course, the lack of clinical data limits the network's ability to address this challenge.

In other cases, organizations have dragged physicians to an end point the physicians do not understand. In these situations, conflict and mutual disdain are likely to emerge. If physicians do not understand the organization's goal, the probability that they will build a supporting culture is nil. To progress to the High-Performing phase, the network must also agree on how physicians will interact, how best practices will be defined and used, how accountable they will be, and so on. These rules of participation generally do not grow organically but are molded by the will of leadership.

Another side effect of lacking a shared vision is low physician morale. Supporting a common goal motivates physicians to engage. Without it, they will focus on individual tasks rather than the big picture. An organization and network with a shared vision tend to retain the physicians they need. Younger physicians especially like the process as they begin thinking about the group in the long run.

Disjointed financial management is another consequence of a lack of shared vision. Physicians focus on their world but generally do not help with the bigger picture. Under risk contracting, this is a huge problem. Getting physicians to understand their roles early, before the network assumes risk contracts, will pave the way to success.

Physician engagement in establishing a ten-year vision has many positive benefits. First, it unlocks the physicians' insights—and doctors have great perspectives because they are closest to the care process—into how to achieve the vision. Second, it unifies them to support the network's strategic priorities. At HSG, we have never been involved in a vision development process that did not make those priorities crystal clear.

The vision can serve as a guiding constitution or a foundational document that helps with day-to-day decisions. At its best, the vision will do the following:

- *Drive physician actions.* We have seen physicians commit to best practices and work with their specialist peers to do the same. The resulting reduction in practice variation has led to better clinical outcomes.
- *Drive physician leadership behavior.* The vision's clarity makes the process of sifting through complex situations and making appropriate decisions much easier for physician leaders and healthcare managers or executives.
- *Drive recruitment and onboarding.* The vision is a document that can be shared with new physician recruits.

By defining the commitment made by both sides, the document tells the recruit exactly what he is signing up for. Healthcare organizations have found it eases onboarding and aids in transitioning new physicians into practice.

LACK OF STRONG PHYSICIAN LEADERSHIP

Physician leadership is at the core of network evolution. In some organizations, lack of physician leadership may be perceived as lack of physicians with leadership capabilities. In reality, physicians may not be empowered to directly contribute or may have poorly defined roles, which is an organizational failure to unleash the physicians.

To ensure a steady supply of physician leaders for the network, organizations need to address four key elements:

1. *Leader selection.* Many organizations apply little rigor to this process, believing that success as a medical staff leader is enough proof of effectiveness and that someone who is politically acceptable is also competent. More consideration should be given to defining the skills and traits required for the position and conducting formal candidate testing. Making leadership selection an open process, with input from a physician advisory group, will further strengthen the selection process.

2. *Leader development.* Development of a leader comes in three forms: education, mentoring, and experience building. Creation of a formal progression process, supported by feedback through mentoring, will help in identifying prepared, qualified, and trained leaders who can navigate complex problems.

3. *Role definition.* Many organizations appoint physician leaders without defining and communicating their roles and responsibilities. If things don't go as expected later,

these organizations wonder why the leaders did not achieve the desired performance and outcomes. Clear definition is particularly important in dyad relationships, which need to be cultivated.

4. *Physician accountability.* Holding physicians accountable is not an industrywide norm. But establishing physician-leader expectations and objectives, engaging a broad group of stakeholders in physician-leader assessment, and giving formal feedback are all part of engendering accountability.

OTHER BARRIERS

In addition to the big three barriers discussed, we frequently see six failures related to the tactics and implementation of employed networks:

1. *Failure in the due diligence process, or poor acquisition.* CEOs rarely meet with a group of admitting physicians that they do not want to work with. Often, an executive's motivation, or simply inexperience, can cause serious problems during the due diligence process. Sometimes, the available practice data are poor, and the organization still might not have all the information just before a contract is signed. When practices are in distress and the organization is motivated to help, even experienced practice buyers can make errors. Those errors can lead to long-term network problems or scare the organization away from logical purchases.

2. *Failure to employ the right doctors.* Building a High-Performing network out of a hodgepodge of physicians is difficult. Failure to strategically target the doctors needed leads to long-term problems. For example, one CEO declined assistance in thinking through the selection of physicians to employ, and he decided to target a

dermatologist as the organization's first acquisition. That selection did not lay the groundwork for long-term success.

3. *Promising physicians that "nothing will change."* This type of promise causes resistance to progress as the network advances to the Operational Chaos phase, and it makes further movement to the right of the growth curve a challenge. If the network is to grow and be effective, almost everything must change.

4. *Operating independently.* More than once, we have witnessed a group leader (usually a physician, because a layperson does not have the power to act in this way) go rogue by pursuing strategies and vision independent of the organization's goals and objectives. The best way to avoid this situation is by jointly creating and regularly reviewing the shared vision and associated strategies. For example, one five-hospital system, with more than 300 employed physicians, was not coordinating its efforts with the employed network. The system CEO, for mostly political reasons, did not insist that the hospital division and employed physician division work together or support each other. The next CEO forced a resolution, part of which included the departure of the physician leader of the network.

5. *Lack of data analytics infrastructure.* Many organizations have installed a single electronic health record (EHR) platform across the enterprise, so sharing information between the organization and the practices has become easier. What remains a big problem is the absence of tools to accurately analyze the EHR data. Managing risk in this environment is very difficult. A lot of venture capital money is being spent on fixing this issue, but many of these fixes are unproven.

6. *Failure to define how the employed network will integrate with private physicians.* Chapter 11 is devoted to this topic,

and it provides suggestions on how to address this failure and how to set clear expectations.

CONCLUSION

This chapter focuses on worst practices in employed networks—practices that can be characterized as failures to plan and/or failures to implement the appropriate plans. The cases at the end of this chapter relate to two universal challenges. The first case relates to the failure to establish a shared vision, and it describes how one system addressed that deficiency. The second case deals with the failure to create a management infrastructure, and it examines the ramifications of that decision for one hospital.

ADDITIONAL RESOURCES

Articles

Barker, N. D. 2016. "Is Your Infrastructure Contributing to Your Physician Network Losses?" HSG. http://hsgadvisors.com/thought-leadership/articles/infrastructure-contributing-physician-network-losses/.

McWilliams, T. R. 2017. "Mastering Dyad Management." HSG. http://hsgadvisors.com/thought-leadership/articles/mastering-dyad-management/.

Online Data

MGMA DataDive Cost and Revenue Survey: www.mgma.com/data/benchmarking-data/costs-revenue-data.

White Paper

HSG. 2018. "Physician Network–Building a Shared Vision." http://hsgadvisors.com/thought-leadership/white-paper/shared-vision-roadmap/.

CASES

The following cases illustrate the concepts discussed in the chapter. The healthcare organizations featured in this section have had a long-term relationship with our consulting practice, HSG, and have given us permission to discuss their employed physician network journey.

St. Claire Regional

St. Claire Regional in Morehead, Kentucky, employs more than 75 physicians and other providers. As the network expanded, a physician leadership group was created with the objective of integrating the various practices and defining the direction of the network. Significant progress was made initially but had slowed and plateaued. The physicians and executives defined a shared vision for moving the network forward over the next decade, and they established strategic and operational priorities that would focus and accelerate the network's evolution.

The St. Claire Medical Group had disparate operational processes, cultures, electronic health records, and levels of accountability. Its leaders believed that variation needed to be reduced and that the network needed to create a common strategic and operational focus, but they were unclear on how to make that happen. The health system chief medical officer sought outside advice from HSG. Our work started with a couple of conversations and expanded to planning the creation of a common vision for the network, with the involvement of the system CEO and group chief operating officer.

Approach
The narrative vision is an aspirational description of how the group will function ten years down the road. The proposed

vision statement was developed by a steering committee consisting of 12 formal and informal physician leaders and four system executives, three of whom were involved in the initial consulting discussions and one of whom was responsible for quality initiatives. This collaborative approach allowed the physicians to assume full ownership of the newly articulated vision. It also created a platform of discussion between executives and physicians.

Aside from the vision, two other elements were addressed. First, an organizational structure recommendation was submitted to formalize the enhanced roles of physician leaders and their reporting relationships within the dyad management system. Second, an outline of key strategic initiatives was developed as a guide to implementing the vision.

The steering committee was asked to consider two primary questions in their deliberations:

1. What does the network need to do to ensure success in a value-based purchasing market?
2. How should the network function to make the doctors proud to be associated with it?

A key step was the presentation of the proposed vision and associated organizational structure to the entire physician network. The physician members of the steering committee delivered the presentation, took ownership of the content, and enthusiastically shared their perspectives on the vision.

The group then split into groups to allow for more intimate discussion and direct feedback. Each small group was facilitated by a physician member of the steering committee. During the breakout session reports that followed, most of the concerns and comments were related to how the vision would be accomplished rather than what it should include. The consensus was that the outlined vision was desirable. In

continued

addition, the executives suggested four initial strategies to pursue, which the group at large considered to be a reasonable start.

The physicians also embraced the proposed organizational structure, even though it eliminated their traditional practice arrangements. They applauded the identification of formal physician leadership positions within the network and, perhaps even more significantly, the newly expanded physician representation in the system's senior leadership: Three physician leaders were added to the CEO's major decision-making body.

Results and Impact

The actions taken by St. Claire's management in concert with physician leaders resulted in a number of positive outcomes:

- They accelerated the evolution of the network to meet the demands of value-based care by focusing the discussion on essential strategies.
- They set a precedent for more collaborative interactions among the physicians and between physicians and administration.
- They instilled the shared vision among the physician leaders, frontline physicians, and executives.
- They provided a road map and a strengthened organizational infrastructure to propel the vision forward.
- They created greater representation for physicians in both group and system operations, with a 300 percent increase in physician representation on the president's council.

The bulk of the vision implementation and execution lie ahead, but both management and physicians agree that the process set the stage for real progress. Each group believes the engagement enhanced its ability to deliver results in a value-based care environment.

Hospital in the Southeast

A 300-bed hospital in the US Southeast engaged HSG to perform an operational assessment of its rapidly growing employed physician network. Leadership was concerned that the network's management infrastructure had not kept pace with its growth. After reviewing the findings, the senior executive team decided to make a change in the infrastructure. We provided interim executive management for the network while conducting a national search for a permanent network executive.

Approach
Within the first two weeks, we had placed a qualified, experienced interim administrator on the ground to stabilize the network. During the first week of the 12-week interim engagement, we met with senior leadership and the interim administrator to outline priority items that needed to be addressed during the engagement. Action plans and timelines were attached to each priority to ensure that these items were addressed and implemented during the duration of the interim engagement. Weekly status calls were held with senior leadership to make sure the timelines were met and to reprioritize action items, if necessary.

Permanent Executive Search
Running concurrently with the interim administrator on-site, we began recruiting a permanent executive for the physician network. To ensure that the search was completed effectively

continued

and efficiently, we held weekly calls with senior executives to review milestones in the search process. After an extensive search and several interviews, five finalists were chosen to take a predictive index survey. From these five candidates, three were selected for on-site interviews with the management team, and one was chosen to lead the network. The permanent executive search was completed within the stated 12-week time frame.

CHAPTER 4

Eight Elements in High-Performing Employed Networks

Important principles may, and must, be inflexible.

—Abraham Lincoln

To develop a High-Performing employed network, you must deliver on eight elements. All of them must be managed and integrated over time. In this chapter, we discuss these elements and the ways they evolve as the network matures.

THE EIGHT ELEMENTS

The sequence in which these elements are presented reflects the sequence in which they must be addressed. However, this sequence does not represent their order of importance. In fact, all eight are important, and all are *required* for high performance.

Strategy

Defining your strategy and creating a shared vision with your physicians are crucial first steps in building a High-Performing network.

Aligning the network strategy with the organizational strategy is also critical, and it starts with the shared vision. When you know where you want to go, it is much easier to develop a road map to get there. As you develop the vision, consider the other seven elements. How are those elements, such as physician leadership and culture, incorporated into the vision?

Next, review the organizational strategic plan. Which elements of that plan require physician-supported tactics, and how can the employed network support the organizational strategy? What is the network's role in making the organization successful?

The network strategy should also address what physicians need to be employed and the geographic locations where they should be deployed. Which physicians do we want in the group and, perhaps more important, which ones do we not want? What specialties are required, and will value-based purchasing and/or population health imperatives change those requirements? What is the ideal mix of primary care and specialty physicians? Should physicians be aggregated to create critical mass? All of these are questions to consider when building the strategy.

The last point about strategy is process oriented. How should physicians be engaged so that they can help develop the plan, thereby gaining their acceptance and support? What is the best way to collaborate to create physician ownership of the final plan? Generally, that process leads to the Physician Advisory Council and its role in the network.

Culture

The difference between a great and an average medical group is culture—the shared values, expectations, norms, and objectives that unify and drive the disparate members of the network to work together. Cultural problems must be addressed, given that employed groups generally start as individual practices, each with its own established set of beliefs and values. A loose confederation of physicians will not produce great long-term collective performance. To get the process moving, explicit discussions on culture should occur at the Physician Advisory Council level. What specific behaviors are required? How should we orient new physicians into the culture? How can we measure culture and incorporate it into the dashboard, using care coordination, access, and other types of measures? Try the open-ended survey questions at the end of this chapter to get the dialogue started.

Quality

Improving care processes and outcomes has never been more important. Networks need to focus on quality to gain physician support because, for physicians, patient care is the top priority. In addition, as reimbursement systems and incentives change, quality-related financial incentives become increasingly important. Your employed group represents your best opportunity to drive the necessary changes throughout the hospital.

Defined broadly, *quality* stands for clinical quality, service excellence, access as part of service excellence, and operational efficiencies. Without strong physician leaders, a shared culture, and dedicated support, groups will make little headway on quality issues. A clear vision statement, defined in the strategy element, helps overcome the natural inertia that results from physicians and practices simply believing that they are doing fine work.

To measure and improve quality, the network needs data. It needs to understand its current performance before it can move on to the next step of setting improvement priorities. Of course, data can be a significant barrier, and most groups do best if they start with simpler, easier-to-measure quality issues.

The network also needs a function for evaluating evidence-based standards. This topic is big, and we have seen groups succeed when they have set a specialty-level objective and rewarded the use of evidence-based standards.

The patient experience issue is tough to tackle. Delivering consistent positive experiences is every network's goal, because it creates satisfied patients and a stronger brand. The challenge comes in making patient satisfaction a priority. In the early years of network development, process improvements that have an immediate impact on the bottom line, such as managing schedules and the revenue cycle, take precedence over the patient experience.

The effect of selecting individual physicians on network quality cannot be overstated. Recruiting the right physicians and acquiring the right practices are essential to building a quality network. An important next step is to communicate the vision and behavioral norms with the new physician recruits and practice acquisitions so that they understand the commitment they are making.

Finally, the network's quality program needs to be built with an eye on payer expectations, which represents the most direct route to wringing value from the network. The long-term goal is preferential treatment from payers, especially self-insured employers. Share your successes with them and make them understand the results being produced and the cultural commitments being made. And make sure your employed physicians deliver the information directly by involving them in interactions with employers and insurers.

Physician Leadership

Physician leaders who understand the big picture (strategy and vision) and can translate it to physician behavior are invaluable. Invest in their development and growth. There are two levels of physician leadership. The first level is the executive, who either is in a dyad management relationship or has sole responsibility for the network. A rigorous selection process and a well-thought-out incentive system for executives are important. Choose someone who is respected by network members and trusted by other executives. The second level is service leadership, who likely will serve on the Physician Advisory Council. Service leaders' support of the strategy and vision are crucial, as is their ability to engage other physicians and capture their insights and perspectives.

In their roles, physician leaders must

- emphasize clinical best practices,
- follow management best practices,
- police bad behavior that may run counter to the culture, and
- be accountable for the network's results.

We want to be clear that these are not medical staff roles. Selection and expectations are different and even more rigorous for physician leaders because, ultimately, they can make or break the network.

Management Infrastructure

Failure to invest in a management infrastructure has created more red ink in employed practices than any other single issue. The network will not perform well without a management infrastructure that includes practice managers, physician leaders, and managers with functional expertise.

Typically, lack of practice managers presents financial consequences in the revenue cycle, payer credentialing, and staff training areas. It is a penny-wise, pound-foolish proposition to economize here. Saving money on practice manager salaries can cost you 10 times more in another area.

The network needs dedicated physician leaders. Compensate them, and create a system of accountability.

Managers with expertise in human resources, finance, quality improvement, information technology, and other functional areas are essential parts of the infrastructure. Hospitals and health systems vary in how they manage these functions, but network resources for addressing financial issues are the most critical for network leaders to control. Financial analytics and the revenue cycle work best when they are not intertwined with competing organizational resources.

Quality improvement can be decentralized, ensuring that the network gets the attention it needs (although creation of silos is a risk).

A robust infrastructure expands the depth of your management team. Rather than treat the network like a department, the organization should treat it like the big business it is.

Aligned Compensation

Physician compensation is, by far, the largest cost in the network. It must be used to align physician behavior with high-performing actions. Compensation is a complex challenge and inevitably evolves with the network. From salaries to work relative value units (RVUs) to clinical quality incentive systems, aligned compensation changes as the network moves right on the growth curve toward the High-Performing phase.

Many errors in compensation can be made. The first is overcompensating and exceeding fair market value (FMV); however, regulations have rendered noncompliance costly. A second error is the lack of a systematic or consistent methodology for compensating physicians. This error presents a management nightmare and makes engaging physician leaders in compensation discussions difficult. A third error is designing compensation plans that fail to address poor performance with reduced pay.

Most discussions focus on physician compensation, but staff compensation is relevant as well. Rather than letting physicians manage patient scheduling, offer incentives for front-office staff to fulfill this responsibility, which would lead to greater practice productivity and better patient access. It will make a big difference.

Brand

Developing a strong brand is generally a longer-term objective. A fundamental question is how the network's brand relates to the organizational brand. Implicit in that statement is a requirement that physician leaders not run off and work on their brand independently. A second implication, which is difficult for many physicians, is developing a single brand for the network. In acquired practices, the practice and its physicians have already built a unique identity and following. They have made a living on the basis of their patients' respect for their brand. Agreeing to be a part of a broader brand is difficult. This obviously has implications for the organization in specialties such as orthopedics, where the institution benefits from the strong following of many loyal physicians.

Another big challenge is the environment within the individual practices. A strong brand strives for network-wide consistency in applying best practices, which can mean massive changes for staff and physicians. This barrier leads many groups to delay this discussion. The lack of management infrastructure makes it difficult to implement in any case.

In the early stages of network development, having a marketing budget and resources can be helpful. Promoting a marketing mind-set in the group can also lay the groundwork for a deeper brand discussion.

Payers and their perception of the brand should be a key consideration. The value of your brand in their minds and the ability of the brand to produce results they need are key. This ties back to our discussion of quality and the importance of sharing positive quality and cost outcomes.

Financial Sustainability

Losses in employed networks are often brought about through the confluence of fast growth, limited investment in management talent, and limited experience managing physician networks. Stemming these losses is essential as groups prepare for the next financial challenge—risk contracting.

The first step in achieving financial stability is putting a management infrastructure in place. The second step is aligning physician compensation. The third step is undertaking an assessment to determine where the opportunities for improvement lie. Benchmarks from the Medical Group Management Association (MGMA) or AMGA can help shed light on those opportunities. Network physicians need to be informed of and understand those opportunities.

A tight, well-managed revenue cycle is one key to success. It involves a lot of basic blocking and tackling, such as working denials, getting good information upfront, and collecting copays.

Building a network that can produce profits by managing care through risk contracting is a longer-term goal. Physician accountability is required. Better data are required. Payer understanding of network capabilities is required. All of these elements must fall into place for success to occur.

A final step in achieving financial sustainability is market power. Having a big group that insurers need gives you leverage. In our experience, controlling 30 to 35 percent of a primary care market gives you leverage. Don't be afraid to use that leverage during negotiations.

A related reality is that you are building something new, something that has not been present in most markets. The data and infrastructure required to manage risk are more expensive than the infrastructure to manage a small practice. Know that some costs will not be paid for in the short term. Make sure your board understands these realities as well.

THE EIGHT ELEMENTS IN THE CONTEXT OF THE GROWTH CURVE MODEL

As networks grow more sophisticated and advance toward high performance, they must adjust the way they handle the eight elements in each phase. For example, the level of physician leadership in a network that is managing risk is different from the level of leadership of a group that is acquiring independent practices as part of a growth strategy. How the elements are addressed in each evolutionary phase (Novice, Rapid Growth, Operational Chaos, Strategic Focus, Value, and High-Performing) are outlined in this section.

Strategy

In the Novice phase, we rarely see a strategy. Network development is sparked by outside stimuli, mostly a recognition that failure to employ physicians hurts patient care or the organization's financial performance. In the High-Performing phase, the strategy addresses care management across the continuum, payer interactions, quality and cost objectives, and value-based care. The path between the two phases is long and complicated.

Typically, networks in the Rapid Growth phase establish a strategy to address labor force issues. They think about systematically targeting certain specialties or physicians. A secondary strategy is to not violate regulatory guidelines, focusing on FMVs and due diligence.

The Operational Chaos phase and the mounting losses it generates necessitate a different take on strategy. The strategic focus turns to management infrastructure and financial goals. In this phase, executives begin to ask themselves how to gain value from the network. Part of the answer is through revenue generation, including the reduction of referral leakage. Another strategic revenue issue is group growth, although mounting losses make executives timid about aggressive growth.

The Strategic Focus phase is when organizations get serious about network strategy. If the strategy has not yet been developed, leaders address the network's shared vision and strategic priorities. Care coordination and best practices become priorities. The team usually focuses on growth in this phase, overcoming the concerns about losses that have slowed this consideration. However, the growth is strategic in nature, focused on primary care, service line expertise, or physician capabilities needed to manage risk. Another area of focus is access. The network recognizes that it can become the organization's front door to services—through both physical locations and electronic connections.

During the Value phase, clinical efforts are focused on value-based purchasing requirements. The network is the locus of the strategy to meet the requirements and gain the related financial rewards. The network also starts experimenting with risk, one-sided accountable care organizations (ACOs), or some direct contracting. It is recognizing that payers are target customers.

The High-Performing phase strategy includes delivering predictable outcomes, predictable costs, and patient access. The network is ready to tackle risk contracting.

Culture

In the Novice network, physicians function independently, with little to no concept of being part of a group. In the Rapid Growth phase, the concept of the network starts to become evident, but little effort is made to foster the culture. Discussions tend to raise basic questions such as, Who is in the group?

In the Operational Chaos phase, the need for a shared culture is becoming clear, but financial realities and lack of management infrastructure delay progress. In the fourth phase, Strategic Focus, culture gets the attention it deserves. Physician leaders are in place and recognize that culture must be established to achieve most anything. Explicit discussions are a staple on the Physician Advisory Council's agenda.

In the last two phases, the culture becomes ingrained. Physicians expect to work collaboratively on best practices, the economics of being in a network, and the network's future direction. Group norms have little tolerance for physicians who do not accept the established culture.

Quality

In the first three phases, networks rarely are successful in addressing quality, although they try. But the lack of management infrastructure, culture, and vision make progress difficult. As groups emerge from the Operational Chaos phase and physician leaders develop, the need for a quality focus becomes obvious. This perceived need is accelerated as the physicians and managers begin to discuss vision. No physician envisions being in a mediocre network that is not concerned with quality. The need for a plan is intuitively obvious.

In the Strategic Focus phase, networks make three leaps. First is a data leap, and the network begins to acquire information to address quality issues. The second is a commitment to group quality objectives, with the Physician Advisory Council leading the charge. The third, which has the most variability, relates to specialty groups' embracing the vision of adopting best practices and acting on that vision. When this happens, quality improvement efforts slowly become more ubiquitous.

In the Value phase, the network applies its new knowledge to value-based purchasing requirements, including those of private payers. It addresses ACO-type deals using the new capabilities. It looks at quality across the continuum of care rather than in silos. A High-Performing network expands and strengthens these capabilities and then integrates them with financial insights, to take another leap forward.

Physician Leadership

Novice groups have no physician leadership, except perhaps from informal leaders who have been employed. Physicians may continue to manage their practices. This approach is sustained through the Rapid Growth phase, although an organizational chief medical officer is likely to start exerting some influence over the network out of necessity.

In Operational Chaos, the need for physician leadership is more apparent as management struggles to gain control of the burgeoning network. Some organizations start the development of Physician Advisory Councils at this point. A part-time physician leader is usually the answer.

As networks move to the right side of the growth curve, starting with Strategic Focus, investment in physician leaders accelerates. It is not uncommon for the vision and strategic plan to call for full-time physician leaders and paying physicians for their time on the Physician Advisory Council. These actions coincide with the realization that the plan cannot be implemented without strong physician leaders.

In the final two phases, physician leadership is in place, ingrained, and influential in organizational decisions. Often, multiple physician executives are present, a recognition that the organization's and network's strategies have evolved to address care delivery.

Management Infrastructure

With Novice networks, the practice manager may stay in place after practice acquisition and report directly to the organizational CEO. This arrangement is the textbook definition of no infrastructure.

In the Rapid Growth phase, the infrastructure relates to acquisitions. A team is developed to address FMVs, due diligence, and other recruitment issues. In addition, at this point, a practice manager for the network is in place. The experience and capabilities of that leader are usually, but not universally, poor.

Operational Chaos creates an environment in which the need for better infrastructure becomes obvious. Organizational executives recognize the need for more talent, although they often do not know where to find the talent. This issue is exacerbated by the reality that the talent pool is not deep. Often, the best talent is a practice manager who has only managed a small group.

By the Strategic Focus phase, the organization is committing to the development of a management infrastructure. The physician leader helps with this task, recognizing the requirement and advocating for it. The practice manager is the second advocate, quickly realizing that more management horses are needed.

As networks enter the Value and High-Performing phases and start managing risk, the need for management with functional skills becomes apparent. Whether housed in the organization or the network, those skills must be acquired.

Aligned Compensation

Compensation can be one of the more vexing problems. Many employed networks have started by paying straight salary but have come to regret doing so, as physician effort declined. Doctors, who had previously made their way by being productive, no longer were driven by productivity. Ironically, many High-Performing networks are returning to pay straight salary—but they have put in place the culture and management controls to allow this approach.

In the Rapid Growth phase, the focus is on recruitment, which generally creates great variability in compensation and can be an operational nightmare. As losses mount through the Operational Chaos phase, the focus switches back to paying for productivity. Work RVUs become the basis for payment to physicians, and this model generally remains, with some adjustment.

In the Strategic Focus phase, incentives may be added, although they may be limited to physician citizenship (e.g., participation in quality improvement, not acting out). Slowly, features are added for achieving quality measures tied to payer incentives or service line objectives—particularly in the Value phase, where the group is focused on quality metrics tied to reimbursement. This phase often has another twist: a limit on productivity compensation for physicians who are not meeting quality incentives. For example, productivity pay may be limited to the 60th percentile unless all quality objectives are met. This motivates physicians to focus on both productivity and quality but punishes practices that churn patients without delivering quality care.

Brand

This element rarely receives any attention until the Strategic Focus phase. In the first three phases, practices tend to retain their identities, although the larger network may develop a name and logo or announce the relationship on signs and letterhead. None of the hard work around the brand—creation of a consistent care process, consistent patient experience, and reputation for results—happens until later in the network's evolution. While some networks may decide against developing a separate identity or brand from the organization, we believe that is a mistake. A strongly branded network can be a health system's biggest asset.

Financial Stability

In many cases, organizations have reconciled themselves to the reality of group finances. Losses are at an acceptable level and are offset by organizational profits. It is normal to see networks drag down the organization's operating margin but not to the extent that executives want to divest the group.

In terms of trends across the curve, we tend to see subsidies mount through the Operational Chaos phase. Subsidies may also grow in the Strategic Focus phase as investments are made to produce strategic benefits from the group. That said, losses tend to stabilize in that phase and trend downward in the Value phase, because of the network's management maturing, physician engagement in the network's financial affairs, and sometimes incentive payments.

Can a High-Performing network make money? Can it manage risk so well that it becomes a profit center? From our perspective, this capability has yet to be proven. Many more mature organizations still experience losses in their physician networks. Part of that reality is how reimbursements are distributed. Organizational executives are more comfortable negotiating hospital rates, so they tend not to spread them out based on where the value is being created. Like most people in the industry, we have a wait-and-see attitude and recognize inherent barriers to profitability in the current reimbursement model.

CONCLUSION

Exhibit 4.1 summarizes this chapter's concepts in chart form. Although this discussion and the exhibit represent what is typical, all networks are unique to some degree. Keep that in mind as you assess your network's performance. The exhibit also makes obvious that your network's evolution toward high performance is not consistent over the eight elements. Physician leadership may be more advanced than your strategy, for example. Such variability is normal. Understanding it will help you think about network priorities going forward.

ADDITIONAL RESOURCES

Article
HSG. 2014. "67 Tips for Developing a High-Performing Physician Network." http://hsgadvisors.com/thought-leadership/white-paper/67-tips-developing-high-performing-physician-network/.

Open-Ended Culture Survey Questions
1. What does it mean to be a medical group physician?
2. What behavioral norms are essential to drive the group's culture?
3. How do we select and onboard new physicians or providers so that they understand the expectations?
4. How will we address group members who are noncompliant?
5. What skill set (including knowledge base) must physician leaders possess to guide this effort, and how do they gain those skills?

Exhibit 4.1: The Eight Elements in Each Phase of the Growth Curve

Eight Elements	Growth Phases					
	Novice	Rapid Growth	Operational Chaos	Strategic Focus	Value	High-Performing
Strategy	Minimal	Focused on growing the group, at times tied to the hospital strategy	Incremental focus on financial performance and supporting management infrastructure	Get serious; define vision for the group and strategic priorities, including quality and access	Focus on quality metrics, payer requirements, and risk-contracting experiments	Robust, integrated with the health system or hospital; focus on payers and risk
Culture	No group expectations	Cultures of acquired groups still dominant	Recognition that common culture is needed	Physician leaders explicitly address behavioral norms	Norms become ingrained and more formal, tied to compensation	Expectations and group norms clear
Quality	Limited focus	Limited focus, except via The Joint Commission	MIPS/MACRA related; energy is on finances	Great focus, better data, and commitment to best practices	Focus on value-based purchasing metrics, one-sided risk, and care across the continuum	Robust; integration of quality and financial insights
Physician leadership	Minimal	CMO getting involved out of necessity	Need for physician leaders more obvious; develop a physician advisory council, and perhaps hire a part-time medical director	Greater investment in physician leaders, often with a full-time physician leader for the group	Greater investment in physician leadership, including formalized development processes	Greater development in physician leadership

continued

Management infrastructure	Minimal investment	Practice manager in place; resources related to practice acquisitions	Greater investment in subject matter experts (such as revenue cycle and quality) and paid physician engagement in management	Dyad in place; many groups upgrade their practice leader to an executive position	Enhanced subject matter experts around risk and population health	Continued enhancement around financial modeling and quality
Aligned compensation	Salary or RVU	Complexity created by varying deals	RVU focus to deal with finances	RVUs plus citizenship and quality incentives	RVUs plus quality incentives that drive reimbursement	Salary in some cases; quality metrics supersede RVUs
Brand	No focus	Develop a group name and logo	Develop a marketing plan	Begin to create consistency in the practices	Further drive consistency in experience and care	Leverage the brand with payers and patients around outcomes and experiences
Financial sustainability focus	Minimal	Initial focus on not creating problems with poor deals	Assessment to define opportunities for improvement	Physician leader's engagement in managing losses	Improvement, some incentive payments related to value-based care	Uncertainty around risk contracting but opportunities for upside

Note: CMO = chief medical officer; MIPS/MACRA = Merit-Based Incentive Payment System/Medicare Access and CHIP Reauthorization Act; RVU = relative value unit.

PART II

Network Growth and Maturity

NETWORKS MOVE FROM the Novice phase to the High-Performing phase in a logical progression. Each chapter in this part of the book—chapters 5 through 10—defines

- the characteristics of the phase and what management experiences;
- the eight elements of an employed physician network, and how management deals with issues associated with these elements; and
- the key areas of focus—what management needs to do to move the network forward.

Cases, recommendations, resources, and practical examples are provided in each of these chapters.

CHAPTER 5

Novice Phase

You can always tell a novice rider: They aren't comfortable in the saddle and have to hang on.

—Harry Carey, Jr.

THE NOVICE PHASE (exhibit 5.1) of the employed physician network evolution can best be described as the period in which no focused strategy for employed providers is yet in place. Novice networks are usually small, with few physician full-time equivalents (FTEs), and consist of a hodgepodge of specialties. In general, the physicians perceive no significant differences between their preemployment and postemployment status. They tend to operate in the same way and use the same resources they had before becoming employed. The only major change is that their practice is more financially stable, as a result of the investment by their new employer—the hospital or health system.

Novice networks exist in markets where the following factors are present:

- Healthy, stable independent practices that are able to address provider recruitment needs with or without support from the healthcare organization(s) in the market
- A medical staff without significant succession planning issues, which would overwhelm the existing independent practices

Exhibit 5.1: The Novice Phase on the Growth Curve

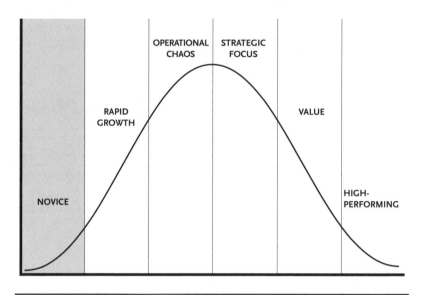

- Little competition between healthcare organizations for providers and provider referrals
- A medical staff culture of independence
- Reimbursement that has not sharply declined or created an economic situation in which independent practices cannot survive

The core characteristics of Novice networks are as follows:

- The healthcare organization does not view physician employment as a core strategy.
- The network is limited in size and scope of specialties.
- Each practice in the network looks and feels independent from the organization.
- Limited infrastructure exists to support practice operations.

If employment is not a core strategy of an organization, then the Novice phase can last as long as the dynamics of the market will support it or until the market shifts and forces the Rapid Growth phase to occur.

WHY NETWORKS INEVITABLY GROW OUT OF THE NOVICE PHASE

A number of factors push Novice networks to enter the Rapid Growth phase, where physician employment begins to become the dominant physician-alignment model.

First, private practices have economic challenges, as costs for staffing, malpractice insurance, and information technology, among others, grow faster than reimbursement rates. Medicare payment increases are minimal at best, and Medicare pay-for-performance initiatives (e.g., Physician Quality Reporting System, Meaningful Use) have the potential to decrease reimbursement if targets are not met. Private insurers are also increasingly aggressive in rate negotiations, and physicians in small practices have no negotiating leverage. Physician income is under significant pressure, and many private practitioners feel powerless to reverse this trend. These financial factors often drive physicians into the arms of hospitals.

Second, the United States is experiencing a physician shortage. Population growth, economic expansion, the aging of the population, and treatment effectiveness that has improved survival rates but led to higher prevalence of illness have all increased the demand for physician services. Some communities lack general internists, as physicians strive to increase their income by pursuing a subspecialty or hospital medicine. Shortages of specialty physicians (e.g., orthopedic doctors) also occur.

Third, more and more physicians desire a balanced lifestyle. The number of hours worked by individual physicians has declined over the years, and younger generations have different ideas and expectations about work ethic and work–life balance. In a busy primary care practice, it is not uncommon for one departing older doctor to be replaced by two younger physicians.

In this environment, hospitals and health systems have to become more aggressive to recruit the type and number of physicians their communities need. In a tight physician supply market, organizations are better able to attract new talent if they offer the opportunity to focus on medicine with the security of a guaranteed income.

THE EIGHT ELEMENTS IN THE NOVICE PHASE

In chapter 4, we introduced the eight elements that must be managed and integrated as the network evolves. A Novice network handles these elements as follows:

1. *Strategy.* The organization's employment strategy at this point may best be described as "reactive." The organization is primarily addressing providers who have approached the hospital and asked to be employed (see exhibit 5.2).
2. *Culture.* No shared or common culture is in place.
3. *Quality.* Formal quality programs are yet to be established. Any quality initiatives that affect the practices are driven by the organization's quality department. The network has limited ability to take on ambulatory-based quality initiatives because of its size and management infrastructure.
4. *Physician leadership.* Physician leadership comes from the organization's medical staff. The network itself has no formal clinical leadership role.
5. *Management infrastructure.* In general, the network management infrastructure is informal or nonexistent. In most cases, management responsibility falls to an organizational executive (e.g., chief operating officer, chief medical officer, vice president of physician services), who

tends to regard the responsibility as just another thing to do within the scope of a larger role. Typically, managers of the private practice are left in place and report directly to the overseeing executive.

6. *Aligned compensation.* Compensation tends to be straightforward: Providers are paid either a base salary or an amount calculated through a simplistic productivity model. Variability in compensation models can create salary administration challenges, however, highlighting the lack of focus on the network by the organization.

7. *Brand.* The network brand either does not exist or is haphazard in its execution. In some cases, the organizational brand is applied directly to the practices; in others, the practices retain their pre-employment brand (i.e., appearance and patient experience).

8. *Financial sustainability.* Organizational executives typically do not consider the network as a big financial concern. Subsidies received by the practices do not significantly affect the organization's profitability. The practices may not even have financial statements, making the subsidies invisible to the executive team. Often, the board is aware of only the highest levels of employed providers and does not consider the network's financial performance as a management issue.

KEY AREAS OF MANAGEMENT FOCUS

In the Novice phase, the network is preparing for future growth and market shifts. As such, it should build a physician employment structure that is as efficient as possible for the limited number of providers in the network. The five key areas of management focus during this phase are discussed in this section.

Exhibit 5.2: Seven Questions to Ask When a Physician or Group Practice Approaches the Organization for Employment

1. Is the physician or group practice part of the organization's strategic plan and vision?
2. Will the physician or group practice help build the organization's market share for Medicare and commercial payers?
3. Are there any concerns with the quality of care provided by the physician or group practice?
4. Is the group practice's current location desirable and/or a part of a strategy (e.g., outreach strategy)?
5. Is the physician's patient volume and productivity declining, stable, or growing?
6. How is the physician viewed by the medical community, and how will his or her inclusion affect the organization's group culture?
7. Does the group practice have any physicians who are viewed as strong leaders?

Key Area 1: Planning Proactively for, Rather Than Acting Reactively to, Growth in Physician Employment

Barring major unforeseen changes in the healthcare landscape, growth in physician employment is inevitable. Prepare your Novice network with the following steps.

Establish a proactive plan for network growth

The major component of this plan is a physician alignment and manpower development strategy. This strategy defines (1) the relationships the organization needs with current providers and (2) the organization's future recruitment plans. By articulating these two things, you will have much of the information needed to start aggressively employing physicians, if and when it becomes necessary.

Look at potential employment needs

Compare your recruitment strategy and strategic goals with the supply of independent private practices in your market. With the organization's support, can existing providers help meet market demands in a way that is beneficial to the organization? Is greater competitor activity anticipated in the market? Are younger physicians willing to join private practices with the incumbent risks? (These issues are addressed in greater detail in chapter 6.)

Maintain strong, open communication lines with core independent physicians

Many executives in organizations with a Novice network believe, "If the practices are happy being independent, we're happy." There's nothing wrong with that sentiment; however, it can easily become an excuse for not informing these core independent providers about the organization's employed network (e.g., how it works, what its future looks like, how providers can join the group). Executives who say, "If they want to be employed, they'll come talk to us," may end up unpleasantly surprised when that same group is employed by a competitor, which made the effort to recruit these providers. The physicians' justified response to this missed opportunity may be, "Well, you never even talked to us about it!" Executives must maintain strong, open dialogue with core independent providers and "take their temperature" regularly about employment opportunities. This way, surprises do not happen and physician alignment does not shift overnight.

Key Area 2: Building Basic Management Infrastructure

Create the foundation for future employed network growth by building a basic management infrastructure that supports the practices already employed. Address the following four issues.

Put the right leaders in place

For most Novice networks, this means evaluating the executive bandwidth and capability to manage the growing network. Once the number of employed physicians reaches a critical mass (about 15+ providers), having a partial FTE in charge of the network becomes a detriment because of the lack of focus and the need to develop an in-depth infrastructure. At this point, on-site managers in practices should be able to report to one member of the organization's management team.

Find a billing solution that fits network needs

Many Novice networks choose one of two lackluster options for billing: (1) maintain billing at the practice level or (2) assign the practice revenue cycle function to the organizational billing office. The practice-level billing personnel may have less incentive to be diligent, given that the practice now has an employed status. The organizational-level billing office may give the practice revenue cycle activities short shrift, given the relative size or amount of dollars. For most networks, the ideal option is to outsource billing to a third party. When the network is big enough to support its infrastructure, billing can be brought back in-house to a practice-only central billing office.

Train the support staff

Adequately train newly employed support staff about the network's business processes, such as supply ordering, charge capture and submission, human resource requirements, and other administrative practice procedures.

Build basic reports and dashboards on network performance

Given their decentralized nature, many Novice networks lack basic reporting capabilities. Running financial, practice-level, and provider-level reports, as well as circulating and explaining them to practice staff and providers, will go a long way toward reinforcing desired behavior. In chapter 12, dashboards and their evolution are addressed in detail.

Key Area 3: Getting Employment Deals Done the Right Way

In the Novice phase, organizations employ physicians reactively as opposed to proactively. Organizations typically spend less time and effort on creating a standard process for employment negotiations or deal making and physician onboarding. The result is a wide array of processes and agreements. Reduce variation in this area by developing a standard process that incorporates the following principles.

Communicate expectations and desires

Providers who are exploring a transition from a fully autonomous, independent practice to an employed, hospital-based entity with significantly less (or very little) autonomy face many hurdles. Early in employment discussions, organizational leaders and the physicians should discuss their motives and desired outcomes. This discussion provides both parties the opportunity to evaluate whether future employment is likely, what points of interest are important to each party, and how they will collaborate to achieve each other's objectives (e.g., quality and productivity goals, timely completion of medical records, timely charge reporting, participation in organizational committees).

Perform practice due diligence

Developing a sound acquisition process that involves true due diligence, fair market value (FMV) determinations, and financial sustainability projections for the organization is key to doing things "the right way." Due diligence ensures the practice has no major operational or quality issues that could become a liability for the organization. It includes reviewing and analyzing the practice's financial statements, historical compensation and production models, payer mix, staffing, contractual relationships, lawsuits and risk management issues, practice management and electronic medical record systems, revenue cycle, and Current Procedural Terminology data. With this information in hand, the organization can make a fully informed decision on whether to continue employment discussions.

Engage currently employed physicians

Performance is not the only factor to consider during due diligence. Determining whether the physician fits with the culture of the employed network is also wise. Having currently employed physicians meet their potential future partners is a good way to gauge cultural compatibility and gives the candidate the opportunity to speak candidly with peers and gain a deeper understanding of what being a part of the network means.

Use a consistent deal-making process

For many Novice networks, employment contracts are a mishmash of agreements with differing structures and variables. This variation happens for several reasons, the biggest of which is the involvement of multiple organizational executives, each of whom uses different deal-making approaches. As a result,

- contract terms are highly inconsistent across employment deals;
- contracts are signed under contrasting views of the practice's strategic importance, which leads to disagreements about the practice's value;
- term lengths vary, which causes surprises and constant pressures at contract renewal time as well as last-minute, haphazard renegotiations;
- fears arise that physician payments are inconsistent with contract parameters; and
- contracts are drafted that conflict with FMV tenets because compliance review was not performed.

Using a consistent process executed by the same team members minimizes variability in contract agreements.

Key Area 4: Being Selective in Employing Providers Who Approach You, and Setting the Right Expectations About Employment

Many networks are plagued for years by the organization's pitch during the Novice phase that "nothing will change" about a practice when it joins the network. Agreements, expectations, and promises during the Novice phase (even when the network comprises just a handful of physicians) will shape the network's culture as it matures. The best way to avoid long-term cultural and performance issues within the network is to employ the right providers with the right expectations about what employment means.

Develop a rubric for selecting candidates

Making the right physician investments depends on developing standards on who you will—and will not—employ when asked. The political ramifications of saying "no" on the front end are much less severe than the potentially lengthy removal of a poorly performing or noncompliant provider down the road.

Involve the same personnel in deal making

All potential providers need to hear the same message during employment discussions. To ensure consistency in voice and messaging, the same individuals should be assigned to the task. Organizations that send different executives to approach provider groups bring variability and confusion to the process.

Lay the groundwork of expected performance early

Use the initial meetings with providers to proactively set basic expectations for physician productivity, availability, record completion, and other "citizenship" requirements as a member of the employed network. As your network grows, laying the groundwork will become more important and will likely lead to better adoption of expectations down the line.

Key Area 5: Educating Key Stakeholders About Future Change

As employment grows as a physician-alignment strategy, all of the organization's key stakeholders—the board(s), leadership and management, and providers—should understand its purpose, what physicians want from employment, and what is required to make employment successful. During the Novice phase, management of the network is not usually a high-visibility effort, but this is a good time to build awareness and understanding of the organization's future.

Educate the board

Especially in the Novice phase, board members question why the organization must support physicians who were previously independent. The simple answer is, if the organization wants to fulfill community needs, it must pursue physician employment. Many younger physicians are not interested in private practice, and the laws of supply and demand mean that doctors can earn more through employment. This type of simple, basic answer will reduce the number of questions in the short term, but it will not build board support for the investment required over the long haul. To provide that kind of understanding and support, you must be proactive and educate your board on the rationale for the physician employment strategy—now and in the future. In constructing a board education initiative, some executives have focused on the following questions:

- What market forces are driving physician employment?
- What operating standards must the organization pursue, and how would they affect subsidies?
- What is the strategic value of the investment in physician practices?
- How does the organization's investment benefit the community?

Do not approach this topic from a defensive position. Use data on physician shortages, practice performance, and the strategic value of your investment. Also, be repetitive. Your board will not absorb all of this information in one sitting, nor will the members remember a discussion from two years ago (they tend to have short memories). A quarterly board report on this topic, tying it to the overall financial health of the organization, will be valuable. (See Miller and Johnston [2018] on how HSG helped Huntsville Health educate its board about its physician employment strategy.)

Educate the leadership team

Educate the organizational and network management regarding the differences between managing a hospital or health system and managing a physician practice or network, as well as the new competencies required. Executive teams also need to get on the same page with their messaging about employment in the organization. One common theme we see in the Novice phase is the negativity felt by executives about employment. They openly make remarks such as, "We don't want to employ physicians," or "We don't like employing physicians," when speaking to the medical staff. This negativity carries forward as the network grows.

Educate the providers

Often, in Novice networks, a generational gap exists in medical staff attitude toward physician employment. More experienced providers who have built independent practices tend to be negative about employment models, regardless of the economics behind them. Some of this resistance will be overcome only with attrition. Make physicians understand that employment is necessary at this point in your network's growth, which will likely ramp up as the organization recruits more providers. Setting this expectation is key to gradually getting physician support for the network's existence and operation.

CONCLUSION

Networks can move quickly from the Novice phase to the Rapid Growth phase. Having a plan in place for how to make that transition ensures the organization's ability to quickly respond. Following are the key learning points of this chapter:

1. *Establish a plan for the future.* Novice phase networks are almost always forced into the Rapid Growth phase. Have a proactive plan for what the next phase will look like and when you think it will occur. Don't respond to this eventuality on the fly.
2. *Build an appropriate management infrastructure for your network's size.* Having a small network is not an excuse to leave it unmanaged.
3. *Use a consistent methodology for acquisition and compensation.* Variability is difficult to manage and results in negative outcomes for all parties involved.
4. *Make smart choices about the providers you are employing now, when your network is still small.* These physicians will help set the cultural tone for when the network is larger.
5. *Educate all of your stakeholders.* Employment is a major cultural and operational shift for hospitals. The learning curve is steep and acceptance takes a long time.

REFERENCE

Miller, D., and L. Johnston. 2018. "Does Your Board Understand Why Physicians Are Employed?" *Becker's Hospital Review.* Published February 22. www.beckershospitalreview.com/hospital-management-administration/does-your-board-understand-why-physicians-are-employed.html.

ADDITIONAL RESOURCE

Miller, D. W. 2018. "Building a Physician Employment Strategy." HSG. http://hsgadvisors.com/thought-leadership/articles/building-physician-employment-strategy/.

CASE

The following case illustrates the concepts discussed in the chapter. The healthcare organization featured in this section has had a long-term relationship with our consulting practice, HSG, and has given us permission to discuss its employed physician network journey.

TJ Samson Community Hospital

TJ Samson Community Hospital is a 133-bed independent community hospital in Glasgow, Kentucky, approximately 90 minutes south of Louisville and 90 minutes north of Nashville, Tennessee.

In 2009, TJ Samson was relatively geographically isolated from major competition. It had a broad and diverse group of independent practices in its market that had historically served the community's healthcare needs very well. It had a total of eight employed providers, a collection of one- or two-physician practices with multiple specialties. These practices were managed by the hospital's Physician Services, and they still had the same branding and operations as when they were independent. Losses on the practices were not measured or reported in any meaningful way. The hospital's medical staff viewed employment negatively, believing it was something providers who "couldn't make it independently" resorted to.

In 2009, competition intensified in the regional market. A large independent medical group from another market started aggressively targeting TJ Samson's core providers, offering employment deals that threw the economics of independent practice out of whack and forcing the hospital to develop a response.

continued

With HSG's assistance, TJ Samson created a comprehensive physician-alignment plan. This plan (1) identified the core providers whom the hospital should proactively target for employment and (2) defined the structural elements required in managing a more robust employed network.

By 2011, TJ Samson's employed network was approaching 50 employed providers.

CHAPTER 6

Rapid Growth Phase

Growth is painful. Change is painful.
But, nothing is as painful as
staying stuck where you do not belong.

—N. R. Narayana Murthy

As NOVICE NETWORKS evolve, they move into the Rapid Growth phase (exhibit 6.1). This is the phase when employment becomes the dominant physician-alignment model. This shift generally occurs for one of four reasons:

1. *Strategic needs.* The hospital or health system has strategic growth needs that cannot be addressed by independent physician practices. The practices are unwilling either to help recruit needed providers or to develop the necessary capabilities within their specialty.

2. *Succession issues.* The organizational medical staff is aging more quickly than the independent practices can absorb and bring in new recruits. Practices at risk of dying out must be stabilized through physician employment, and the employed recruits must be placed in those practices to transition them.

3. *Competitors seeking alignment with organizational providers.* As competitors seek to grow their patient volume and geographic footprint, they disrupt traditionally

noncompetitive markets with their physician-alignment activities. If your system anticipates aggressive behavior by a competitor, employment of your traditionally independent (yet loyal) physicians is a likely outcome.

4. *New physicians' desire for employment.* Most physicians coming out of residency today want to be employed. Strong independent groups may mitigate this trend in some markets, but recruitment and employment are mostly synonymous. Recruitment is not a priority for many organizations that are still in the Novice phase, and they also tend to struggle with succession issues.

The core characteristics of Rapid Growth networks are as follows:

- Employment is the organization's dominant physician-alignment model.
- The physician market is shifting from independent to employed, resulting in a sudden, significant increase in employed providers.

Exhibit 6.1: The Rapid Growth Phase on the Growth Curve

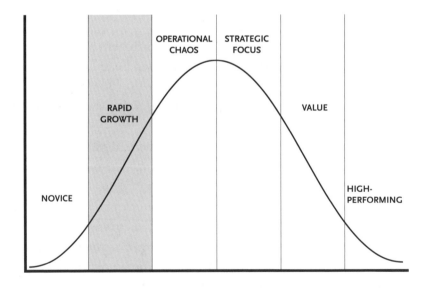

- Growth in employed networks and full-time equivalents becomes the measure of success, regardless of who is being brought in.
- Management bandwidth or capability is focused on getting deals done and ensuring strategic goals are met—to the detriment of network operations and management.
- The management infrastructure of the Novice network feels massively inadequate for the needs of the rapidly growing network.

As the organization's focus on employment shifts, more and more providers jump on the employment train, and the network begins to grow exponentially.

Networks typically remain in the Rapid Growth phase until one or both of the following events happen:

1. Most physicians in the market are employed by the organization or a competitor. The remaining independent providers are "the ones who will stay that way" (although this is not always the case).
2. The organizational board and/or executive team, sensing the network is getting large and the financial commitment is getting unwieldy, begins to pull back on executing the employment strategy.

Either of these events sends the network into the next phase—Operational Chaos—in which the network's management, daily operations, and financial performance come under intense scrutiny, and the network experiences pressure to improve its performance.

WHY RAPID GROWTH BECOMES OPERATIONAL CHAOS

As many networks that have evolved from the Novice phase to the Rapid Growth phase can attest, the number and frequency of employment deals made amid this transition are significant and far beyond what the organization anticipates. Late in the Rapid Growth phase, a common refrain among executives is, "How did we end up with all of these employed providers?" An organization may start its employed network journey by focusing on recruiting new physicians out of residency, but the increased emphasis on employment tends to draw interest from the market's independent providers, even those on the record as "fiercely loyal" or "never going to be employed."

When an organization starts employing providers in earnest, it sets off a cultural shift—fast in some markets, slow in others— that makes employment an easier consideration for the physicians. Employment becomes a way out of staffing issues, electronic medical record (EMR) acquisitions, management challenges, and diminishing payer reimbursements. An "everyone else is doing it" mentality brings providers who want to evaluate their options to the executive team's door. That employed physicians are better compensated than are their independent counterparts is obviously a draw as well. This leads to a difficult-to-navigate dynamic in which the organization is not only proactively making deals with its core providers but also being approached by other physicians who now want to explore opportunities for employment.

Once this strategic and cultural shift occurs, deal making or employment negotiation gets fast and furious. The deluge of physicians approaching the organization, and vice versa, causes three issues that eventually lead to operational dysfunction:

1. Executive teams work off different scripts as they meet with providers. This inconsistent messaging results in variation in understanding about what employment will mean, how providers will be compensated, and what will change in the practices.
2. Management time is spent on "getting" the providers instead of figuring out how to integrate them. This focus results in frustrating operational challenges as soon as the physicians join the network.

3. Network resources are quickly overwhelmed, and cutbacks are made to things that should not be cut (e.g., credentialing, onboarding, revenue cycle, staffing). This drives overall network operations into a state that requires constant "firefighting" just to survive from day to day.

Once Rapid Growth slows, the network begins its transition to the Operational Chaos phase.

THE EIGHT ELEMENTS IN THE RAPID GROWTH PHASE

A rapidly growing network handles the eight elements of an employed network as follows:

1. *Strategy.* Without some form of a physician alignment and labor force development strategy in place, an organization cannot effectively be proactive in its recruitment or acquisitions strategy (see exhibit 6.2) and will remain in reactive mode. Strategy in the Rapid Growth phase should focus on prioritizing physicians in the market according to organizational goals. Which providers are core to the organization's overall strategy and service line–specific strategies? Which will drive volume to meet market share targets? Which will help meet value-based performance goals? If the network does not have this kind of plan in place, the Rapid Growth phase is the time to develop one.

2. *Culture.* A common culture and vision are usually not present in this phase. They are not even management priorities for the network.

3. *Quality.* At this point, the network is not focused on program-based quality activities other than the basic activities the practices were already performing before employment (e.g., participation in the clinically integrated network or other quality initiatives).

4. *Physician leadership.* Given the priority on growth, formal physician leadership does not usually exist early in the Rapid Growth phase, unless the leader is the organizational chief medical officer or chief clinical officer.

5. *Management infrastructure.* The infrastructure is limited in the Rapid Growth phase. As the number of providers grows, the problems associated with this lack of management infrastructure become apparent. Physicians have to be onboarded, staff members have to be hired, and systems have to be connected. This is the point at which the executive in charge of the network starts looking for a network manager. The result is often disappointing and does not solve the many issues the network is experiencing. The network manager then becomes the chief firefighter but has neither the bandwidth nor the experience to move the network forward in a meaningful way. Practices still continue to largely operate independently, but with a bit more direct oversight and input from the organization. As financial performance of the network worsens without a remedy in sight, the need for a stronger management infrastructure becomes crystal clear.

6. *Aligned compensation.* During Rapid Growth, providers' pay often takes a backseat to getting the deal done, which leads to an array of compensation arrangements with differing terms and degrees of fair market value compliance. Physicians end up with the compensation model that is simplest to negotiate, not the one that best aligns incentives. By the end of the phase, physician compensation administration has become a major issue because of the inconsistencies in the contracts and compensation models.

7. *Brand.* In most cases, this phase is when the network gets its first real name (e.g., Health System Physician Group, Health System Physician Partners). This brand tends to exist on paper more than in practice, however.

8. *Financial sustainability.* At the start of the phase, as the employment strategy begins to broaden, the financial focus is the effect on the organization (e.g., What will happen to our bottom line if we lose or don't employ these providers?). Later in the phase, as the employment strategy matures and more physicians are on the payroll, the financial focus shifts to the effect on the network (e.g., Why are we losing so much money on our employed network?).

Exhibit 6.2: Strategic Considerations in Physician Acquisitions

Hospitals are acquiring physician practices at a brisk pace. Driven by the economics of medical practices, shortage of some physician specialties, and various other issues, the trend toward physician employment is growing. In helping dozens of hospitals evaluate acquisition opportunities or complete acquisitions, we at HSG have seen almost every scenario imaginable. The situation that causes the biggest concern is when organizations react to an opportunity rather than think through its strategic implications. At best, these organizations spend time and valuable resources without gaining any real strategic advantage. At worst, they create long-term problems by acquiring nonproductive practices.

Ideally, organizations should develop an employment strategy that addresses the specialties the organization wishes to include in the network; the vision for the culture, behavior, and performance of employed physicians; and the infrastructure that helps make the strategy a success. With that strategy defined, organizations increase their chances of producing the desired results and developing an employment model that meets their objectives.

In evaluating an acquisition, you must consider six sets of questions:

1. **Does the practice fill a strategic need?** Is the specialty necessary to implement a service line growth plan? Does the acquisition help the organization expand into a new geographic market? Does the acquisition increase the organization's leverage with insurers? Does the acquisition support another element of

continued

Exhibit 6.2: Strategic Considerations in Physician Acquisitions (continued)

the strategic plan? If you cannot answer yes to one of these questions, the acquisition might not be appropriate.

2. **Does the practice fill a community need important to the organizational mission?** Does the acquisition bring new expertise to the organization, improve patient care, or help provide coverage and consults?

3. **Does the organization have the capital resources to sustain the acquisitions strategy?** Although the acquisition may be very logical, it could be a bad strategy if it limits the organization's ability to pursue other opportunities. In addition to the acquisition costs, ongoing subsidization must be considered as well. These issues should be addressed in the strategic plan or employment strategy. An associated financial plan will help you better understand the overall financial implications of pursuing the acquisition of a practice. Failure to understand the financial implications before making the deal is one of the biggest omissions.

4. **Will the physicians fit the organizational culture you are developing?** Will the physician work well in a larger organization? Will the physician support the objectives of the organization? Will the physician work to develop a team approach to tackling priority issues? These are crucial questions if you want to avoid selecting a problem doctor. If your network has a Physician Advisory Council, this is a great discussion for that group.

5. **Does the organization have the infrastructure needed to make this acquisition a success?** Some acquisitions can overwhelm the acquiring organization's management capabilities and systems. Does the organization have adequate leadership, information technology (IT) capabilities, and billing systems to make it work? Does the compensation system create appropriate incentives? All of these must be answered before an acquisition is completed, and corrective actions must be integrated into the financial plan.

6. **Can the employment model be replicated for other practices?** Practice negotiations can be intense, and physician demands vary greatly from group to group. It is crucial to consider what

precedents you are setting and what problems you are creating
for the people who will have to implement the deal. Although
100 percent uniformity is impossible, it is strategically important
to minimize variation—because variation will have operating
and political costs in the future.

As you consider an acquisition, use these questions to prevent
problems. Better yet, develop an employment strategy by asking
these questions in a planning process *before* you begin acquisitions.
Doing so will help you avoid wasting scarce resources and ensure
that your employment efforts are successful and meet the strategic
objectives of the organization.

KEY AREAS OF MANAGEMENT FOCUS

During the Rapid Growth phase, the employment strategy is executed as efficiently and as consistently as possible. Given the speed
at which markets transition and the limited executive bandwidth,
the plan will not be implemented perfectly, but limiting the dam-
age done now will make the Operational Chaos phase less painful.
The five key areas of management focus during the Rapid Growth
phase are discussed in this section.

Key Area 1: Executing a Proactive Growth Strategy

In the Novice phase, the first key area was "Planning Proactively for,
Rather Than Acting Reactively to, Growth in Physician Employment." In the Rapid Growth phase, this key area gets vetted again
and recalibrated, now that employment growth is a reality in the
market. To execute this plan, network management should follow
these recommendations.

Revisit the growth plan

Now is the time to look at the plan again and define the following:

- What specialties do we need to employ on the basis of organizational strategy?
- Which specific practices do we need to target and in what order?
- Where does recruitment into employment fit into our strategy, and over what timeline?

Take a hard look at the strategic value of potential acquisitions

In the Rapid Growth phase, organizations can fall into the trap of approaching their most closely aligned independent practitioners first. These are the doctors who participate in medical staff leadership and who are called on first when a committee has an opening for a clinician. We advise maintaining an open dialogue with these providers, but they should not be the first acquisition targets during this phase. Many executives find it difficult to separate likability and close relationships from strategic value. Take a step back and reassess who is truly valuable from a strategic perspective. Then, home in on those physicians, rather than approach the easygoing conversationalists first.

Get out there and approach providers

One of the biggest challenges in moving from the Novice phase to the Rapid Growth phase is the management team's reluctance to talk with providers about employment. In addition to the obvious cultural barriers, there is the specter of doubt among executives, who may think, "I don't know what I'm talking about, so the providers are going to pick me apart," or "If I talk to them, I may create demands that are not currently on their mind." Although very understandable, these fears must go by the wayside. Now is the time to get aggressive in your recruitment and employment strategy.

Key Area 2: Developing Consistency in Deal Making or Negotiation

In the Rapid Growth phase, as the organization employs providers faster than ever before, one of the biggest challenges is achieving consistency in deal making. Multiple executives talk to a diverse group of providers, each with a different need or want, in a relatively short time frame; different contracts get put together in the name of getting the deal done. In the very short term, fast negotiations may be regarded as a win, but as the challenge of administering these agreements emerges, much angst and regret over the deals arise. To combat this issue, we recommend the following steps.

Establish standards for deal making
It is hard to quickly come to a standardized agreement when providers are transitioning to employment en masse, but all parties benefit from predefined employment standards and contracts.

Form a physician transactions committee
Once a week, convene those in charge of deal making to review ongoing negotiations and provider needs and wants as well as to discuss what is tolerable for the health system from financial and management bandwidth perspectives. Check potential deals against the deal-making standards. This committee of deal makers should understand who is being approached, why the deal is advantageous, how the contract terms meet the standards, and what the challenges are to completing the deal. This committee should also ensure that the acquisitions are not creating compliance problems.

Create a standardized due diligence and operating assessment process
Employing providers is the focus in this phase; buying and operating a practice are not. For two factors that are so interlinked, they

are remarkably distinct in this phase. Develop a standardized due diligence and operating assessment process. This process defines what the organization will be acquiring and what management challenges will need tackling when the practice is brought into the network.

Key Area 3: Controlling the Message in the Medical Community

Manage the organization's relationship with independent physicians. Going through the Rapid Growth phase will not lead to employing every key provider or practice in the market. These groups of continuing-to-be-independent providers will remain an important part of the organization's future, so don't take them for granted. Instead, invite them into the tent, so to speak, and show them that employing doctors does not change what team anyone is on.

Physician education and input into strategic growth should be used as tools to help align the independent providers with the goals of the employment strategy. However, be mindful that, for these independent providers, watching most of the market move toward employment (while they stay put) can be alienating.

Key Area 4: Balancing Infrastructure Development with Growth Goals

During Rapid Growth, infrastructure is almost, by definition, an afterthought. Providers are recruited into employment and/or acquired at a much faster rate than the network management infrastructure can be built. This makes the Operational Chaos phase inevitable. However, although the next phase cannot be avoided, it can be mitigated by the proactive decisions made during the Rapid Growth phase.

Reinforce the organizational chart

A dedicated executive leader for the network should be put in place now. Unfortunately, this role is often overlooked because the network manager may be hesitant to bring another person into the decision-making structure or add another cost. However, an executive leader can be immensely valuable as more physicians are employed and integrated. Again, it is so important to be proactive when entering the Rapid Growth phase. Having a team in place allows the network to not get bogged down in day-to-day issues and to stay in front of the challenges that will inevitably occur in the Rapid Growth phase.

Invest in a common information technology solution

As Rapid Growth progresses, the network will likely accumulate a variety of EMR platforms. The goal should be to get all the practices on a single EMR platform. The speed with which the network makes a decision on this matter depends on the following factors:

- Does the organization have a long-term inpatient and outpatient IT solution in place?
- Is the organization evaluating a change in EMR platforms in the near future?
- Does the organization's inpatient platform have an ambulatory platform that is viewed positively by providers?
- Do most of the acquired practices share a common platform?

In general, we advise against making a hasty decision. The IT selection process should include input from as many providers as possible. Dealing with operational headaches from multiple platforms in the short term is preferable to dealing with long-term provider dissatisfaction with a hasty IT decision.

Temporarily outsource the revenue cycle function

The best arrangement at this point is to use a third-party billing vendor, and then bring billing back in-house once network growth slows and operations stabilize. Many of our clients have used their hospital revenue cycle infrastructure and team to do the professional service billing for their employed physician networks. Some have done so successfully, but most have not, losing hundreds of thousands of dollars in the process. Often, we find issues with workflow and manpower—too many claims and too few people to be effective. Hospital billing and EMR systems with a physician practice module have frequently been a source of frustration as well.

If executed well, in-house billing is likely 1 to 2 percent more cost-effective than outsourcing. But chasing that revenue during the Rapid Growth phase is being pennywise and pound foolish. Billing is a function that can go really wrong, really quickly and result in poor network financial performance and frustrations from providers who got it right before they were employed.

Key Area 5: Recruiting, Acquiring, and Onboarding Physicians Effectively

In the Rapid Growth phase, management bandwidth for successfully acquiring or recruiting providers is put to the test. Executing deals efficiently and effectively—not just getting providers to sign on the dotted line but doing so consistently—is a challenge that requires much forethought and ongoing coordination.

Given that networks enter the Rapid Growth phase from the Novice phase, one of the key questions is, Who is going to do all of this work? While your competitors are recruiting your key independent providers, who in your organization is out there meeting with the providers and making deals? Little to no infrastructure exists for most Novice networks, so this challenge frequently falls to the already busy executive leaders, who are forced to scramble to respond.

But the process of getting providers into the network does not stop once the recruitment or acquisition is complete. Effective physician onboarding is a critical step in successfully transitioning to the network. A lot of networks lose focus on this step. Onboarding failures can result in negative financial outcomes and adversely affect provider satisfaction from the very beginning of the employer–employee relationship.

To proactively address some of these challenges, we offer the following recommendations.

Evaluate management bandwidth and capabilities

Organizational management teams often realize they lack some skill sets and a few capable people to get the work done. This realization leads to one of two outcomes: (1) Executives take on the work of rapidly growing a network as part of their regular responsibilities, or (2) executives quickly recruit or promote team members and then try to get them up to speed as quickly as possible, adopting a "building the plane while flying it" mentality. The traps to avoid here are as follows: (1) leaders getting involved when they do not have the time to be involved and (2) leaders promoting staffers who do not have the skill set or experience to be in management roles.

Define recruitment or acquisition roles and processes

When the Rapid Growth phase hits, it is tempting to take an all-hands-on-deck approach and start sending executives and managers out to talk to providers and execute deals. However, an established process that involves designated team members produces better outcomes and less variation. Define who will be involved in each of the following areas of your recruitment or acquisition process:

- *Workflow.* Who performs what part of the process?
- *Identification.* Who is identifying targets? Who is talking to providers to gauge interest?
- *Engagement.* Who is contacting interested physicians? What message is being conveyed?

- *On-site visits.* Who is meeting with physicians?
- *Deal making or negotiation.* Who is crafting offers? Negotiating deals?
- *Administrative onboarding.* Who is getting providers ready to work? Is there a tight process for getting new providers credentialed or recredentialed with payers?
- *Collegial onboarding.* Who is integrating physicians into the network? What is the process?

Define your onboarding programs
Administrative onboarding is the introduction to operational processes as well as practice logistics (e.g., space, equipment, staffing, IT training). This onboarding should be directed by an administrative leader and the existing practice manager. Collegial onboarding, on the other hand, focuses on the seamless integration of the new provider into the network, the organization, and the community. This onboarding should include both personal (e.g., communities, schools, other resources) and professional (e.g., tours, logistics, culture, peer relationships) elements.

Develop a 100-day onboarding plan for every provider
The 100-day plan should encompass time and activities before the physician's start date and during the initial couple of months after hiring. This plan will include dealing with operational or administrative and cultural issues. The key areas to include are as follows:

- Credentialing, licensing
- IT systems and training
- Clinical consults, tests, and support for patient care
- Human resources
- Productivity, quality, and work expectations
- What it means to be part of the group

Every organization has unique requirements, but some of the most common concerns to be identified in a 100-day onboarding plan are as follows:

- Managing physician credentialing, both for medical staff privileges and payers
- Setting dates and assigning accountability
- Establishing expectations for productivity, behavior, culture, and patient care requirements to avoid misunderstanding
- Identifying the key professional relationships that need to be put in place to help the physician practice effectively
- Assigning each new physician a physician mentor from within the organization to ensure integration into the culture and operational hierarchy
- Setting expectations regarding going out into the community and meeting other members of the network and medical staff
- Assigning responsibility to practice staff to ensure the physician is ready on day one
- Assigning responsibility to the front desk team to create a scheduling template so that patient scheduling is handled appropriately
- Developing an orientation schedule for the new physician that includes department managers, nursing leadership, and key physicians within the hospital departments

CONCLUSION

The following are the key learning points of this chapter:

1. *Be proactive about strategically targeting providers.* Determine which specialty or physician is strategically valuable; do not simply target those with whom you are most comfortable. Focusing employment efforts on physicians who are already aligned with your organization will not help you execute your strategy.

2. *Promote consistency in deal making.* Create standards for deal making that guide your executive team's actions and ensure as much standardization in employment models as possible. Dealing with variance down the road is a severe political and strategic headache.

3. *Communicate at the executive level.* Start a forum, such as a physician transactions committee, to facilitate communication among executive team members. Prevent multiple executives implementing their own strategy with their own set of rules.

4. *Engage everyone, not just your targets.* Your medical community needs to hear what is going on; quell rumors, which run rampant at this stage.

5. *Think proactively about the management infrastructure.* Don't be afraid to overinvest in people or infrastructure when you know your network will grow significantly. Being proactive now is a lot cheaper than playing catchup later.

6. *Take onboarding seriously.* An imperfect onboarding program is infinitely better than the absence of such a process. It should include a clear designation of duty and authority for integrating employed providers into the organization in an effective and efficient manner.

CASES

The following cases illustrate the concepts discussed in the chapter. The healthcare organizations featured in this section have had a long-term relationship with our consulting practice, HSG, and have given us permission to discuss their employed physician network journey.

Six-Hospital System in the Midwest

A system in the Midwest was struggling with decentralized decision making in its physician network. With no system-level plan in place, executives at the system's six hospitals were implementing different physician recruitment or alignment strategies that did not support the organizational strategic vision. In addition, a limited centralized physician network management team was being asked to manage a growing network with no plan for the network's growth, leaving them chronically underresourced, resulting in increasingly poor network financial performance.

Approach
HSG assembled an overall planning committee comprising system-level executives and physician leaders, as well as representatives of senior leadership and physician leadership from each hospital in the system. Working with this committee, HSG facilitated a comprehensive, system-level physician strategy that focused on the following:

- *Geographic growth.* The primary, secondary, and tertiary markets for each hospital were divided into "strategic clusters." Each cluster's development was prioritized on the basis of market share goals, demographic attractiveness, drive time, and other criteria.
- *Primary care.* The system's primary care presence and access points were evaluated and compared against those of the competition in all markets the system served. A gap assessment was conducted to facilitate the development of a primary care growth plan.

continued

- *Service lines.* Agreement was reached on the system's core service lines, and development plans for each service line were created. Specialties outside those service lines where strategic thought was needed were identified.
- *Advanced practitioners.* Goals for using advanced practitioners across various specialties were standardized, and an advanced practitioner integration development plan was created for each hospital.
- *Physician alignment, acquisition, and recruitment.* A three-year, comprehensive plan was developed that defined growth in primary care and specialty providers from alignment, acquisition, and recruitment.
- *Physician network management infrastructure.* Based on the Physician Alignment, Acquisition, and Recruitment Plan, the gaps in the infrastructure affecting the ability to manage the client's overall physician network at the system level were assessed.

Results

This process generated a coherent, consistent, system-level strategy with buy-in from all hospital stakeholders. A year into implementation, the system is seeing a coordinated effort from hospital leadership in executing a physician strategy consistent with the system's strategic goals. In addition, the physician network has been able to proactively scale its infrastructure, resulting in fewer operational challenges than would normally have occurred with this type of rapid growth.

Hospital in the Southeast

In 2009, a 175-bed hospital in the Southeast had a largely independent physician base and a handful of employed physicians.
There was no alignment strategy to guide its relationships
with either group. With HSG's assistance, the hospital grew
the employed group from 8 providers to 40 over a three-year
period. The resulting downstream revenue turned a –2 percent
margin in 2009 to a +4 percent margin in 2012.

However, as gains from downstream revenue from retained
referrals leveled off, the hospital recognized the need to achieve
additional value from the group to help offset the losses being
generated by practice operations. In addition, as the employed
group grew, independent physicians in the community felt
increasingly isolated and at odds with administration.

Approach
HSG facilitated a planning process that involved hospital leadership, independent physician leaders, and employed providers. This group discussed common challenges in the market,
how they could help the hospital address its strategic and
operational challenges, and how to recruit new physicians
into both independent and employed practices.

Results
A common plan was defined and gained buy-in from the representatives of both physician cohorts. As a result, the employed
and independent physicians had a better working relationship,
and the hospital was able to jointly leverage these groups to
tackle physician-driven initiatives, such as quality and cost
performance improvement.

CHAPTER 7

Operational Chaos Phase

*Anything you build on a large scale
or with intense passion invites chaos.*

—Francis Ford Coppola

IN THE OPERATIONAL Chaos phase (exhibit 7.1), the employed physician network has outgrown the capabilities or capacity of the infrastructure initially established to manage it. This healthcare organization–based infrastructure includes the following:

- Director-level manager whom the organizational CEO assigned to oversee the network
- Billing system
- Electronic medical record (EMR)
- Support functions (e.g., finance department)
- Informal organizational structure, with no clear lines of communication or network chain of command

In addition, during the Operational Chaos phase, physician practices in the network experience the following:

- Rapidly escalating practice costs while reimbursement stays flat

- Dwindling generous deals (deals that are typical during the Rapid Growth phase, in which organizations focus on "getting" the provider and not on managing the losses)
- Layering of organizational benefit structures and overhead onto the practices
- Skyrocketing subsidies

These and other operational issues may cause organizational leadership and/or the board to question the viability of physician employment as a strategy, pull back on employment deals ("We can't afford to employ more providers"), cut network staff or fail to resource management appropriately, and ask already busy executives or managers to take on more responsibility within the network (leading to other problems within the healthcare organization).

Because of these dynamics, Operational Chaos is a dangerous phase. When practice-level financial losses start affecting the organization-level bottom line, the board starts getting curious,

Exhibit 7.1: Operational Chaos Phase on the Growth Curve

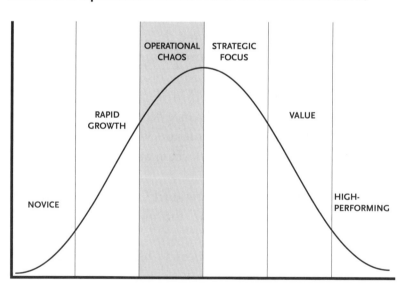

and leadership teams start getting frustrated and anxious. Providers start feeling the pressure, especially when they weren't losing money before.

The core characteristics of a network amid the Operational Chaos phase are summarized as follows:

- The network has grown exponentially from the flurry of deal making, recruitment, negotiations, or acquisitions happening in the Rapid Growth phase.
- The management capabilities of the network have not scaled in the same manner, however, resulting in a mismatch between group size and management resources.
- Current network managers feel the need for day-to-day firefighting as operational challenges seem to spark every day.
- Financial losses are rapid and cause much anxiety, which drives the pullback from the employment strategy and investment in building the management infrastructure.

Networks evolve from Rapid Growth to Operational Chaos when they start to mature and when the organization switches its focus from growing the network to "stop losing so much money on the network." This phase does not have a natural end point. The network will remain here until the organization makes a conscious decision to fundamentally change the way it manages the network. This includes building the right infrastructure, engaging the providers, creating an integrated network, standardizing practice operations, and standardizing compensation arrangements. To leave this phase, the organization must work toward leveraging the group as a strategic asset.

THE EIGHT ELEMENTS IN THE OPERATIONAL CHAOS PHASE

A network in the Operational Chaos phase handles these eight elements of an employed network as follows:

1. *Strategy.* Strategy shifts from growth to management—that is, how do we strategically move every aspect of the network's operation (essentially, all of the eight key elements) forward?

2. *Culture.* Culture development tends to lag behind, partially as a result of management's operational focus, which doesn't allow the time for activities related to vision or culture development.

3. *Quality.* Quality is usually not a focus, either. In most cases, the development of a robust quality program and integration of performance measurement into compensation is a Strategic Focus phase initiative.

4. *Physician leadership.* Engaging providers in the work of network leadership begins in the Operational Chaos phase. To truly address operational and financial performance issues, provider input and buy-in are heavily needed. However, most networks find that physician engagement entails more than inviting doctors to the table. Major cultural barriers must be broken down, and the right type of forum must be developed to solicit appropriate provider input.

5. *Management infrastructure.* The network must build the infrastructure to support the current size of the network. That infrastructure must be optimized to help make the network financially sustainable.

6. *Aligned compensation.* Compensation is ideally standardized. Networks that have gone through the Rapid Growth phase invariably end up with a variety of provider agreements or contracts. Many of these agreements are geared toward what providers want, rather than what the organization needs.

7. *Brand.* Brand is still not a major focus. But at this point, some thought should be given to letting the public know that the organization and practices or physicians are now on the same team. True brand development, however, still takes a backseat to getting the operations right.

8. *Financial sustainability.* Along with establishing an infra-structure, financial sustainability is another core focus in the Operational Chaos phase. The hard work directed at employing providers has resulted in an unsustainable financial position, which may continue without significant intervention.

KEY AREAS OF MANAGEMENT FOCUS

Actions in the Operational Chaos phase should focus on one overall goal: Get the network to a point of sustainability—of financial performance, provider satisfaction and retention, and management satisfaction and retention. Achieving this goal requires developing and executing a plan that will take the network to the next phase—Strategic Focus. The seven key areas of management focus in the Operational Chaos phase are discussed in this section.

Key Area 1: Reorganizing and Rightsizing the Management Infrastructure

To define the appropriate management infrastructure, we ask the organization the following seven questions:

1. Do you have the right organizational structure to effectively manage practices in the network?
2. Are you in the optimal legal structure to maximize revenue and operating efficiencies?
3. Does the practice executive have the skills and capabilities required to implement your vision for the network?
4. Do you have distinct functions and dedicated resources—such as information technology (IT), finance, and revenue cycle—that support the group's day-to-day operations?
5. Do your management capabilities and skill sets reflect the size of the network?

6. Does your IT infrastructure provide your clinicians the clinical data they require to deliver high-quality care?
7. Does your IT infrastructure provide the financial reports and data required to effectively and efficiently manage the practices?

Put in place the organizational structure

The first focus should be on the organizational chart (see exhibit 7.2 for a sample). If you haven't done so, now is the time to appoint dedicated full-time administrative and clinical leadership for the network. The intensity of these roles will vary by network size and other factors. Adequate physician leadership for smaller networks may be 0.2 full-time equivalents (FTEs), although networks with 30 to 40 providers often require full-time medical leadership.

The central billing office (CBO; discussed in key area 4) also needs to have full-time leadership. If practice billing is done through the CBO, dedicated resources are needed to ensure that collections for the practices are accurate, timely, and in accordance with a standardized process.

IT resources need to be brought into the network. At some point, the network will begin consolidating EMR platforms or moving en masse to a new platform. Either way, resources need to be in place to enable or assist with this transition, train providers and staff as quickly as possible, and actively optimize IT use in daily practice.

Review the network's legal structure

During the Novice and Rapid Growth phases, the network is treated as just another department under the organization's tax-ID number. However, this comes with a handful of downsides, most notable of which is that the practices take on the benefit structure of the typically richer hospital or health system that employs them.

With the need to consolidate the many tax IDs under the network, the organization must now evaluate whether moving the network into its own tax ID, either as a for-profit or a nonprofit, makes sense. The financial advantages of switching benefit structures

Exhibit 7.2: Sample Organizational Chart for a Network Moving Through Operational Chaos

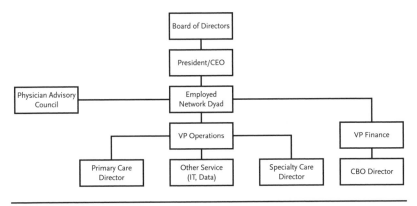

Note: CBO = central billing office; IT = information technology; VP = vice president.

are huge. The core challenge to changing the legal structure is that staffers who perform the same functions (general administration, for example) for the organization and the network will end up with different benefit structures depending on where they work.

Key Area 2: Installing the Right Administrative and Clinical Leaders

Building the right infrastructure starts with getting the right leader in place. This leader is rarely the person who has been in charge of the network through the Novice and/or Rapid Growth phases. Whether your network has gone from 5 to 45 FTEs, or 50 to 500, it needs a skill set now that was likely not present when you started.

Identify the right administrative leadership
To identify whether the current practice administrator in the network is suitable, ask the following distinguishing question first: Do the physicians work through operational challenges with the administrator, or

do they reach out to the organizational executive team to intervene? Engagement of the executives indicates weakness at the practice level.

Next, establish a formal leadership title for the role. Depending on your network's setup, this title may be *executive director, president,* or *vice president* of the network. Some organizations use *president,* to create equal status with the hospital presidents. Regardless of title, this leader can be brought into your network if you treat this search with the same care and importance you give to the recruitment of an organizational executive:

- *Take the time.* Conduct a national search of experienced executives. Done correctly, this search could take 80 to 100 days to complete.
- *Spend the money.* Experienced network leaders typically have advanced degrees and/or certifications. Be willing to offer executive-level salaries and benefit plans to attract and sign the best candidates; this talent pool is narrow.
- *Use the right eyes.* People who have run large networks know inherently what to look for in a candidate. An in-house recruiter or staff from the human resources department may lack the knowledge to evaluate candidate resumes or ask the right screening and interview questions.

Identify the right clinical leadership
Develop a clinical leadership position that functions as part of a management dyad with the administrative executive. For most networks, this role is ideally filled internally, rather than through an outside search. During the Operational Chaos phase, this position is usually part-time, with a goal to introduce aspects of dyad management to the network.

Institute the dyad management approach
Dyad management consists of one clinical member (typically a physician) and one administrative member who co-lead the network. It is a team-based approach in which the physician leader leverages her

strengths and expertise to oversee clinical functions and the administrator brings his strengths and expertise to manage the business operations. Each dyad leader directly contributes to organizational performance through well-defined, mutually supportive individual and shared responsibilities. The exact roles and responsibilities of each leader vary according to the size and complexity of the network, the organization, or the assigned subunit. See exhibit 7.3 for an example of these roles and responsibilities.

Exhibit 7.3: Dyad Management Roles and Responsibilities

Shared	Physician Leader	Administrative Leader
• Developing or implementing strategy and associated action plans	• Providing provider supervision – Performance review – Discipline – Recruiting, onboarding	• Developing operational goals, priorities, and responsibilities
• Fostering group culture	• Creating, implementing, and monitoring clinical practice guidelines	• Monitoring group financial functions—budgeting, accounting, and reporting
• Promoting, monitoring, and reporting group and individual performances – Quality of care – Patient safety – Patient experience – Operational efficiency – Operation budget	• Driving population health management initiatives	• Managing and developing human resources consistent with organizational guidelines, established contracts, and legal requirements
• Developing internal and external organizational relationships	• Evaluating clinical outcomes (effectiveness and efficiency)	• Coordinating necessary support functions—marketing, IT, and financial
• Optimizing clinical informatics and data analytics systems	• Supporting administrative leader	• Supporting physician leader

The development of dyad management usually occurs after the Operational Chaos phase, but this should not preclude the network from beginning to build the approach into its culture.

Key Area 3: Standardizing and Streamlining Operational Performance

Operational consistency—use of standardized measures and approaches to minimize practice variation—is essential, especially during this phase, and should be assessed for the following practice components:

- *Financial performance.* In general, how close to established benchmarks are the losses on each practice? What is the target for losses?
- *Revenue cycle performance.* Whether managed by a CBO or the practice billing function, is the revenue cycle performance in line with or above benchmarks?
- *Staffing levels.* Are staffing levels consistent with production levels?
- *Provider production.* Are physicians producing at the levels expected?
- *Advanced practice professional use.* Do the practices employ nurse practitioners, physician assistants, and other advanced practice professionals? Are these providers, including the physicians, performing at the "top of their license" (Moawad 2017)?
- *Provider compensation.* How does compensation compare with production levels? Are there compliance issues with any contracts due to compensation?
- *Overhead costs.* Are the nonlabor or administrative costs within the practices appropriate?

As you perform this assessment, look at both the individual practices and the trends across the network as a whole.

In general, operationally chaotic networks tend to be operationally inconsistent and are characterized as follows:

- Higher-than-benchmark practice losses
- Poor revenue cycle performance, particularly in charge capture and documentation
- Wildly variable staffing levels
- Wildly variable provider utilization, with some practitioners functioning as nursing staff and some carrying their own patient loads
- Variable productivity, and compensation levels that are not consistent with production levels
- Initially lean overhead costs that balloon as the network progresses along the growth curve (In the Operational Chaos phase, organizations rarely fully allocate to the practices the costs of the management structure. Therefore, as cost accounting systems for the practices improve, overhead costs tend to increase.)

Key Area 4: Formalizing the Revenue Cycle Process

Revenue cycle management is complex and involves a long list of activities (exhibit 7.4). It is affected by stagnant or declining reimbursements, the implementation of electronic health records, evolving local-carrier determinations, and payer credentialing. The emphasis on healthcare fraud and abuse and on compliance has elevated the importance of accurate data reporting and claims filing. The efficiency of a practice's billing operations has a direct effect on the practice's financial performance.

During the Novice and Rapid Growth phases, networks often outsource the practices' billing function under the rationale that it is too important to not do correctly but requires much attention while the practices are amid acquisition. The Operational Chaos phase is the time to bring revenue cycle management back into the network as part of the expanded management infrastructure.

Develop a CBO

The exact setup of a CBO varies from network to network. We recommend evaluating a CBO on the following eight key factors:

1. *Leadership.* Does the CBO have a dedicated, full-time leader?
2. *Roles and responsibilities.* Do the CBO staff members have clear day to-day responsibilities?
3. *Dashboard.* Is a dashboard report generated for key performance indicators? The ability to measure allows network management to make timely and appropriate interventions.
4. *Fee schedule.* Are the fee schedules updated yearly, when the Medicare fee schedule is released? The schedule should be set as a percentage of Medicare reimbursement that ensures the maximum allowable capture from commercial payers (200 to 250 percent). Otherwise, the network is missing revenue opportunities.
5. *Policies and procedures.* Are policies and procedures in place for fee schedule updates, reconciliations, write-offs, insurance follow-ups, denial management, and other functions?
6. *Net revenue collections.* Does the network calculate this metric to get an accurate picture of the CBO's performance?
7. *Appropriate workflows.* Are workflows, such as payer checks and balances as well as coding audits, in place and well defined? Are accountabilities assigned for these workflows?
8. *Staffing.* Is the CBO's staffing level appropriate for the network's size and productivity? Do not try to save FTEs in this area.

Key Area 5: Engaging Providers in Network Operations and Performance

Formally engaging providers in the network's performance represents a shift from past approaches whereby the physicians were engaged

Exhibit 7.4: 21 Daily Activities in Revenue Cycle Management of an Employed Physician Network

1. Patient pre-visit or call for appointment
2. Patient record entry in the EMR
3. Patient check-in
4. Visit documentation
5. Potential charges recorded on a superbill
6. Visit coding
7. Patient checkout and copay collection
8. Posting of the charge
9. Preparation of the day's batch, and checking for missing tickets, hospital reports, etc.
10. Billing office verification of the charge and information
11. Scrubbing of the bill
12. Electronic and paper transmission of the bill to the patient
13. Preparation of the documentation, if necessary
14. Preparation of the explanation of benefits for appropriate posting of the payment
15. Preparation of the patient check for deposit
16. Posting of the payment to the correct patient
17. Review and preparation of any denials
18. Getting additional information for denials from the billing office
19. Resubmission of the claim
20. Working the aged accounts receivable
21. Sending the patient statements

in practice or individual performance. Engagement should focus on developing and building out the network's Physician Advisory Council (PAC). Following are tactics for forming and operating a PAC.

Articulate the purpose

PACs take on many names (e.g., governance councils, leadership councils, boards [informal]), but their purpose is the same: to create a core group of physician leaders who assist network administration with problem solving and strategic direction. Management's message should be as follows:

- We want our physicians to take ownership of the performance and success of the network.
- We need physicians' help and leadership in (1) discovering operational challenges, (2) developing the solutions, and (3) supporting the implementation of those solutions.

Determine the PAC composition

Ideal PAC composition varies according to the network's size and complexity. Provider membership should be relatively inclusive to do the following:

- Achieve the broadest input during PAC deliberations
- Effect the greatest buy-in for the PAC's decisions
- Be representative of the network's specialty mix; geographic locations; provider age or generation, experience level, and gender; and advanced practice professionals mix

In addition, the council should include a member from a newly acquired practice.

The PAC's size must balance inclusiveness with a workable decision-making process. Most councils are led by dyad management (an administrator and a medical director). Other administrative team members are involved on an ad hoc basis, whereas certain ex officio leaders hold positions as standing members; exhibit 7.5 provides a sample PAC composition.

Define the duties

The PAC should be assigned the following responsibilities:

- *Soliciting strategic and tactical input from direct care providers.* Early, ongoing physician involvement in the strategic planning process drives more positive results. Engage your PAC in strategic initiatives related to the network and the organization.

Exhibit 7.5: Sample Physician Advisory Council

Chairs		
Executive director (1) Medical director (1)		
Employed Network Providers	**Employed Network Administration**	**Hospital Executive Leadership**
Physicians (7–9) Advanced practice professionals (1–2)	Operations (1) Finance (1)	CEO (1)

- *Reviewing practice performance.* Performance and metrics should be reviewed through a dashboard format on a regular basis. This review provides the council with the opportunity to replicate positive practices and identify potential areas for improvement.
- *Presenting potential new initiatives.* The PAC is an excellent place to vet proposed initiatives arising from management or the practices.
- *Promoting physician ownership of practice functions and initiatives.* Abdicating this important responsibility will result in subpar performance.
- *Educating and grooming future physician leaders.* Council membership introduces prospective physician leaders to the organizational perspective and strategic objectives. It promotes a collective rather than an individual focus.

Set expectations

All PAC members should be informed of and should embrace membership expectations and ground rules. Consider adopting the following guidelines:

- Assume a fiduciary duty to the system and to peers. Membership does not represent an opportunity to advocate or pursue private agendas.

- Exhibit respect for all those involved in the council.
- Attend meetings faithfully.
- Actively prepare for and participate in meetings.
- Serve as an information conduit between peers.
- Champion PAC-approved projects and initiatives.
- Openly discuss opinions during meetings, but rally behind the final decision.
- Leave what is said in the meeting at the meeting.
- Share PAC discussion feedback with practice members.

Key Area 6: Standardizing and Optimizing Compensation Methodologies

In the Operational Chaos phase, provider compensation is a typical concern for organizational executives and managers. Varying levels of compensation are the direct result of the multitude of deals made during the Rapid Growth phase. When viewed in the aggregate, these deals had different compensation methodologies, incentives, term lengths, agreements for oversight of or working with advanced practice professionals, and compliance complications; lacked alignment with organizational strategic goals; and disregarded other organizational arrangements signed with network physicians (e.g., professional services agreements, call coverage agreements, medical directorships). Building the right compensation plan is imperative at this point.

Get a handle on physician agreements
After Rapid Growth, network providers likely have multiple contracts with one organization, some of which may no longer be relevant. The Operational Chaos phase is the time to make sense of these contracts. Review the contracts or agreements for the following:

- The terms are aligned with the network's strategic goals and objectives.

- Total compensation is within the bounds the organization is willing to pay.
- The fair market value and commercial reasonableness of total compensation from all sources are in compliance with Stark and Anti-Kickback laws.

We recommend these steps: First, conduct a comprehensive inventory of these contracts. Second, compare the total compensation against benchmark to identify concerns about fair market value. Third, compare the terms with organizational objectives. Last, build a plan of action that addresses the following: What changes need to be made? When do contracts expire? How will we educate providers on the needed changes, and how will we get their buy-in?

Strive to align compensation and productivity levels

Financial challenges will drive you to align compensation levels and work relative value units (wRVUs). To start this process, run a comparison of percentile compensation and percentile production. It is reasonable for compensation and production to vary within a +/–10 percentile point range. Consider the scatter diagram in exhibit 7.6; you may use such a diagram to plot your providers' levels or data. Exhibit 7.7 shows the details of this diagram. As exhibit 7.7 shows, the northwest corner of the plot is your biggest concern. These physicians are being paid more than their production can justify. Using such a tool, you can identify what is at risk and what intervention to take for your network.

Start educating physicians

Inform physicians now that compensation changes will be coming, and begin their education on the new methodology. In most markets, this education is focused on transition to value-based reimbursement and includes

- the Merit-Based Incentive Payment System as part of the Medicare sustainable growth rate fix;

Exhibit 7.6: Scatter Diagram: Production vs. Compensation

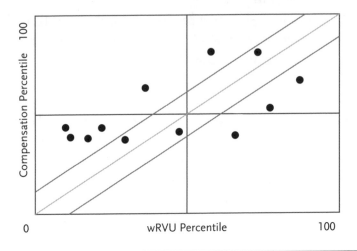

Note: wRVU = work relative value unit.

Exhibit 7.7: Scatter Diagram Data: Production vs. Compensation

High compensation and low production • Not financially sustainable? • Compliance risk? • New/ramping up? • Providing other services?	High compensation and high production • Overworked? • Quality at risk? • Ideal?
Low compensation and low production • Is the physician part-time? • Is there a role for a physician at that level? • Is the physician covering her own costs? • Can we cover our overhead?	Low compensation and high production • Are we at risk of losing highly productive physicians?

(y-axis: Compensation Percentile, 0 to 100; x-axis: wRVU Percentile, 0 to 100)

Note: wRVU = work relative value unit.

- hospital-based programs, such as value-based purchasing and penalties for readmissions and hospital-acquired conditions;
- voluntary alternative payment models, such as value-based accountable care organizations and Medicare shared savings programs; and
- bundled payments.

Your overall message to physicians should be simple: In the near future, our compensation framework will

- gain physician buy-in and ownership;
- support the development of a cohesive culture within the group;
- offer incentives for improvements in productivity, quality, patient satisfaction, citizenship, clinical processes, and teamwork;
- maintain correlation between individual physician compensation and performance;
- be competitive in the national marketplace while considering unique challenges within the market;
- be financially sustainable; and
- provide a consistent foundation that will enable the network to adjust revenue streams as value-based reimbursement models become more prevalent.

Key Area 7: Managing the Relationship with Organizational Stakeholders

Take a step back to (1) look at the impact of the growth in employment on the rest of the organization and then (2) determine where this critically important structure of the employed network fits within the organization's long-established management hierarchy.

Vestiges of how the organization managed provider relationships before physician employment tend to linger. Executives, service line leaders, and other management team members may take offense when key providers begin reporting to the new management structure. Joint planning and focusing on how the group supports the organizational strategy will help address many of these challenges.

CONCLUSION

Following are the key learning points of this chapter:

1. *Force yourself through Operational Chaos.* It's a phase that doesn't go away on its own. Organizations move beyond it when they commit to building the capabilities to manage the network they enlarged during the Rapid Growth phase.
2. *Find the right leaders.* Networks cannot move out of the Operational Chaos phase with only part-time organizational executives or unqualified practice managers. Likewise, a dearth of physician leaders will slow progress.
3. *Do a formal assessment of each practice within the network.* What is working, and what is not? What's the plan for fixing it? What is driving the issues across multiple practices?
4. *Build revenue cycle capabilities.* Make sure this function meets the network's needs, and make sure the network gets paid for what it does.
5. *Start engaging providers.* Lay the groundwork for the expansion of provider leadership, and ask physicians to start thinking about how the network gets out of the Operational Chaos phase.
6. *Start the conversation about compensation.* Deals that were created during the Rapid Growth phase may not serve the network's long-term needs.
7. *Bring your organization's stakeholders along as you work on the network.* Everyone needs to understand why the network requires so much attention and resources.

REFERENCE

Moawad, H. 2017. "Practicing at the Top of Your License." *MD Magazine.* Published May 3. www.mdmag.com/physicians-money-digest/contributor/heidi-moawad-md/2017/05/practicing-at-the-top-of-your-license.

ADDITIONAL RESOURCE

Barker, N. D. 2018. "From Operational Chaos to High-Performing: The Right Path for Your Physician Network." HSG. http://hsg advisors.com/flipbooks/operational-chaos-high-performing-right-path-physician-network/.

CASES

The following cases illustrate the concepts discussed in the chapter. The healthcare organizations featured in this section have had a long-term relationship with our consulting practice, HSG, and have given us permission to discuss their employed physician network journey.

Health System in the Northeast

After a multiyear effort of growing its employed physician network, this health system had a collection of employed physicians, but the network did not function like a group in any sense of the word. When the system retained HSG, the network had

continued

- primary care, specialist, and hospital-based physicians under different tax identification numbers;
- practices with dissimilar names and branding;
- on-site managers reporting to different hospital vice presidents;
- billing done by system staff or by a separate physician billing department on two different systems;
- different compensation models and structures; and
- no group culture or no feeling among physicians that they were a part of a larger unified network.

The system wanted to form a subsidiary organization for the employed physicians that would function under the system's influence but would be managed separately by physician practice administrators rather than system executives.

Approach

For two years, the system added new practices and transitioned existing employed practices into the new entity. During that time, a central billing office (CBO) was established specifically for physician practice professionals and technical services. An electronic medical record, integrated with the practice management system, was implemented in practices. Directors of primary care and specialty practices were hired to oversee practice operations. The entity installed its own chief administrative officer, billing manager, credentialing coordinator, and director of finance and accounting. The practices have been branded similarly and are clearly identifiable as a part of the system's employed physician group. Physician compensation models have been implemented with similar values and structure.

Result

Today, the system's employed physician network is advancing toward being a multispecialty group. The network has an infrastructure, trustworthy data and information, and more provider cohesion and direction. More work is being done to create a shared purpose, vision, and culture.

Apex Medical Group

Apex Medical Group is a not-for-profit healthcare system with facilities in six counties in the Southeast. It employs 140 providers in 19 specialties. Apex sought to optimize its revenue cycle operations to address internal structural factors that were financially affecting the organization. The leadership also was determined to standardize its processes and establish financial accountability and consistency of metrics across its clinics.

Approach

Apex engaged HSG to guide and execute a comprehensive revenue cycle redesign. This redesign involved evaluating historical data, consistently following revenue cycle indicators, implementing a daily budgeted volumes report, creating a dashboard, reorganizing the CBO structure, resolving an insurance denials backlog issue, standardizing a fee schedule, and developing a staffing tool.

Key focus areas of the project included increasing accountability and visibility of metrics across the revenue cycle; therefore, HSG initially provided full-time managerial support to streamline communication and transparency between the CBO and the different practices. The team collaborated to reestablish communication lines between the various points of contact.

Apex's leadership developed a list of key financial indicators that required monthly analysis, established priority when

continued

analyzing these indicators, implemented a revenue cycle meeting structure, and allowed staff to work toward financial goals. In addition, Apex identified revenue leakage to improve the annual net revenue, aided by a CBO now organized around the revenue cycle process (including insurance verification, coding and charge posting, claims processing and payment posting, insurance follow-up, and self-pay collections). The insurance denials were streamlined, and all coding and charge entry staff members changed their work location to the CBO and started reporting to the coding and charge entry lead.

Process documentation, fee standardization, and staffing and productivity benchmarks were all addressed.

Results

Exhibit CS7.1 shows performance improvement, from the third to the fourth quarter of 2016, in all major measures. These results were produced with the addition of eight FTEs and the reassignment of 14 individuals within the network. Annual collections improved by more than $7 million.

Exhibit CS7.1: Third-Quarter vs. Fourth-Quarter Performance

	Q3	Q4
Quarterly collections	$15.84 m	$17.58 m
Net collection rate	90.2%	99.1%[1]
Days in AR	45	40
Denial percentage	3.33%	2.3%

[1] This rate reflects some "catch-up"; expect 2017 to be 96.5%.
Note: AR = accounts receivable; m = million.

Compensation Planning for a Tertiary Hospital

A tertiary hospital on the Atlantic Seaboard with more than 1,000 beds, a children's hospital, a level-I trauma center, and one of the nation's largest transplant centers employs a broad range of specialists—from primary care physicians to transplant surgeons. The compensation methodology for these employed physicians was not consistent across specialties or even within a specialty, and it largely used a base salary model that did not incorporate bonuses for productivity or quality. The hospital was experiencing unnecessary practice losses because of lack of productivity, and it was dealing with an administrative nightmare of reconciling the different types of physician contracts each month and each quarter.

Approach

With HSG's guidance, the hospital formed a steering committee composed of the executive team, board members, and physician leadership. This committee received education regarding industry trends in compensation planning, economic incentive alignment, and financial stability and compliance considerations. Group discussions led to the identification of four key issues that the new compensation plan must address:

1. Program sustainability
2. Quality and productivity incentives
3. Flexibility to expand quality incentives as reimbursement environment changes
4. Fair market value–compliant total compensation package

Next, term sheets were developed that incorporated these components in the structure of the compensation agreement.

continued

These term sheets were reviewed and approved by the employed physician group.

Results

By using a process that incorporated key stakeholder education and direct physician involvement in the creation of a compensation methodology, the hospital achieved a greater level of buy-in from the employed network as a whole. Today, this compensation methodology is applied to both new provider contracts and existing contracts as they expire.

CHAPTER 8

Strategic Focus Phase

In the midst of chaos, there is also opportunity.

—Sun Tzu

WITH GROWTH-RELATED OPERATIONAL challenges better addressed, the employed physician network turns its attention toward the Strategic Focus phase (exhibit 8.1). Specifically, network providers and leaders are focused on (1) building a shared strategic vision and culture and (2) making strategic changes to the network to improve its performance and position it for the future. The foundation for the following goals is set:

- Discarding the collection-of-practices mind-set for the multispecialty group mind-set
- Becoming physician-led and professionally managed
- Aligning providers' objectives with the network's future direction
- Separating from providers who are underperforming or are poor cultural fits
- Developing population health management capabilities

To accomplish these goals, the network must prioritize physician engagement and leadership.

Exhibit 8.1: Strategic Focus Phase on the Growth Curve

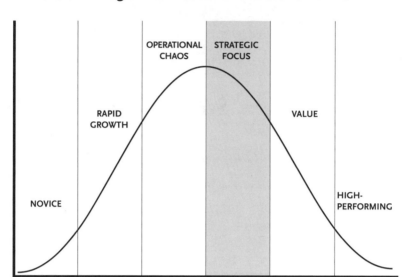

The core characteristics of a network in the Strategic Focus phase are as follows:

- Operations have stabilized as a result of the right-sizing of the management infrastructure and the development of practice management competencies.
- Physicians are engaged in leadership roles, strategic planning, networkwide initiatives, culture and vision work, and other strategic decisions and activities.
- Only providers or practices that are relevant to the overall strategy are recruited and added to the network.
- Weak or underperforming physicians or practices are identified and potentially removed from the group.

The amount of time spent in the Strategic Focus phase varies widely from network to network. In the worst cases, networks

128 *Employed Physician Networks*

struggle to engage providers, who are frustrated with and distrustful of administration. In ideal cases, administration keeps providers engaged, preparing them to move on to the Value phase.

THE EIGHT ELEMENTS IN THE STRATEGIC FOCUS PHASE

A network in the Strategic Focus phase handles the eight elements of the employed network as follows:

1. *Strategy.* Provider engagement and cohesiveness have at last matured sufficiently to make networkwide strategic planning a reality. Together, the strategic plan and strategic vision create a road map for the network's future.
2. *Culture.* The culture is starting to take shape, creating a sense of unity among providers that is essential to achieving strategic goals. However, physicians most likely have not given much thought, let alone discussed, the cultural elements desired for the network. Exhibit 8.2 offers tips to prompt such a discussion.
3. *Quality.* Use of quality metrics, reporting and documentation of quality outcomes, and monitoring of quality data, among others, are networkwide expectations.
4. *Physician leadership.* The network actively begins (or continues) establishing formal physician leadership roles and responsibilities within the network to drive change.
5. *Management infrastructure.* Systems and processes for quality, clinical data analytics, population health, and other functions are established to support the network's strategic plan and help with the achievement of strategic goals.
6. *Aligned compensation.* Compensation plans begin to change to support the organization's strategic initiatives.

Compensation evolves beyond base salary or individual production-driven models to incorporate focused measures and incentives that align provider and organizational initiatives.

7. *Brand.* Defining a common, identifiable brand becomes a core focus in this phase. This brand must represent the network's culture and vision, unifying the look and feel of the diverse practices.

8. *Financial sustainability.* Financial sustainability is no longer the all-consuming issue. By this phase, operations should be stable enough for the losses to decrease.

Exhibit 8.2: Five Questions to Prompt Culture Discussion Among Network Physicians

1. **What attributes of a group make you proud to be a part of it?** This question starts to make abstract concepts concrete by asking for the specific features that providers find valuable about being in a network.

2. **What does it mean to be a group physician?** The answers directly reflect perceptions of the network's current or desired culture.

3. **What behavioral norms are essential to drive the group's culture?** Ask the question directly to get a targeted response.

4. **How will we address group members who are noncompliant?** Holding fellow members accountable is a necessary element of an effective group. Enforcing compliance is difficult. Openly discussing and collaboratively developing mechanisms to promote adherence to group norms and address recalcitrance not only reflect transparency but also elevate collegiality.

5. **What skill set, including knowledge base, must physician leaders possess to guide culture building, and how do they gain those skills?** Leadership characteristics and behaviors are often overlooked during culture discussions. Directly addressing this area ensures a more comprehensive approach to desired group dynamics.

KEY AREAS OF MANAGEMENT FOCUS

After years of fighting fires, management in the Strategic Focus phase has an opportunity to centralize the network's resources and build a vision for the future. This includes shaping the culture, defining a strategic plan, and ensuring the network's infrastructure and compensation incentives evolve to fit its future direction. The five key areas in this phase are discussed in this section.

Key Area 1: Developing a Shared Strategic Vision

The day-to-day challenges of the Operational Chaos phase should be over at this point, but that does not mean the network is ready to move forward. The next challenge is to get the individual practices and providers out of a semiautonomous mind-set and have them begin thinking and acting as a group. Physicians often have a good understanding of how a group needs to evolve to thrive. They understand how they could better serve patients. They understand how variability in care represents an opportunity to improve. They understand why physician leadership is crucial to meeting organizational and patient needs. This awareness needs to be melded with industry and organizational direction, and the vision should be developed for the long term (five to ten years).

Typically, this process results in the following:

- A common definition of "success" for the network (How will we know we are doing well—or not doing well?)
- Improved working relationship between the network providers and the organizational leadership, because common expectations have been identified
- A forum for building stronger relationships between the network and independent providers in the market
- Networkwide service standards for all providers

- A common definition of "access to care" among providers
- Acceptable behavioral standards for providers
- Agreement on how the group's progress toward value-based care capabilities should evolve

A strong, shared group vision, defined with physician leaders, will help propel the development of a strong group culture. The vision also helps ensure the culture aligns with the requirements for enterprise success.

Following are steps to developing a shared strategic vision:

1. Interview stakeholders to understand their perspectives on what the network needs to be in the long term. Focus on group aspirations and perceived problems.
2. Review the organizational strategy for elements that translate to the network.
3. Assemble a group of formal and informal physician leaders and task it with defining the network's ideal or projected state, strategic priorities, or activities in five to ten years. Share with this group the insights and information gained from the interviews and strategy review (steps 1 and 2), as well as market trends.
4. Draft a vision document that describes the common aspirations in some detail. This draft tends to be three to four pages long, leaving less to the imagination so that all physicians can understand its intent.
5. Engage the group in revisions. Developing the vision is an iterative process. Be patient as the group works through edits for about three meetings, focusing on the content, presentation, and clarity rather than wordsmithing. Invariably, the physicians will identify something that is near to their hearts and that reflects a sense of service to their patients. The points of interest and emphasis may change with each version as the group internalizes the content. The revision process increases their sense of ownership.

6. Present the draft statement to the entire physician group. Physician leaders should conduct this discussion. Inevitably, frontline physicians will add further insights, leading to greater ownership.
7. Establish the final vision statement.
8. Review the vision on a regular basis. Make the review part of an ongoing management control system. At least semiannually, the vision statement should be reviewed with two questions in mind:
   - Has a change in the market occurred that generates additional insights or affects our vision?
   - Are we prioritizing the correct strategies?

The core strategies the network must pursue become obvious during the vision process. Those strategies feed into the strategic plan process, which not only makes the vision process tangible but also shows physicians how specific actions tie directly to the vision.

Key Area 2: Creating a Strategic Plan

Strategic success for employed networks is highly dependent on physician buy-in and participation in the execution of the strategies that emerged from the vision process. In a market with increased accountability, your network's future hinges on its physicians' ability to deliver better, more efficient care and to manage to metrics. Engaging doctors to gain their understanding of the market's trajectory, insights into how to respond, and support for strategic initiatives is critically important. The strategic plan should be a logical outgrowth of the shared strategic vision process described in the first key area. If the vision is the *what*, the strategic plan is the *how*.

A strategic plan's content varies from one network to the next, depending on the priorities and aspirations defined during the vision process. However, a strategic plan has common components, such as the following priorities identified by an HSG client during a strategic planning process for its network:

1. Empowered physician-led advisory board to guide the network and make key decisions
2. Care processes based on best practices and an infrastructure to institutionalize those standards
3. Processes that facilitate patient hand-offs, thereby improving care across the continuum
4. Robust primary care strategy, including the medical home model
5. Integrated electronic health record across the network
6. Referral system that keeps patients in the network
7. Common brand and marketing strategy
8. Regional growth strategy
9. Compensation structure that aligns incentives across the network

Key Area 3: Expanding the Role of Physician Leadership

The role of the Physician Advisory Council (PAC), established during the Operational Chaos phase, should be expanded in the Strategic Focus phase to further engage network providers and encourage physician leadership. This expansion includes the following tasks:

- *Evaluate the composition of the PAC.* As the network grows and evolves, the PAC membership must reflect the composition of the network to ensure fair representation of providers. Thus, a methodology for evaluating the PAC composition should be established.
- *Form subcommittees to operationalize the PAC.* Subcommittees not only perform several key functions but also, and most important, create opportunities for provider involvement and reinforce the concept that network-related work is not strictly for administrators or executives. We recommend four subcommittees: (1) operations and finance, (2) clinical informatics, (3) quality, and (4)

advanced practice professionals. Exhibit 8.3 is a sample PAC subcommittee.

An additional comment about advanced practice professionals is in order. In most networks, advanced practice professionals are indispensable, especially in primary care. Creating a formal subcommittee composed of these practitioners recognizes their importance and gives them a voice in the network structure.

Use a dyad management structure
If one does not already exist, a clinical leader needs to be appointed as a formal member of the network's management team. This role functions

Exhibit 8.3: Sample Physician Advisory Council Subcommittee Structure

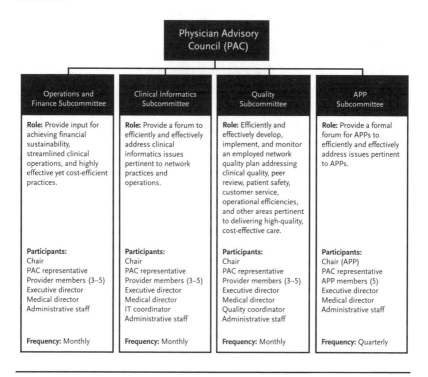

Note: APP = advanced practice professionals; IT = information technology.

in a dyad or co-leading relationship with a network administrator (see chapter 7 and exhibit 7.3 for a fuller discussion of dyad management). Instituting a dyad management structure immediately injects physician leadership into the formal management hierarchy and engenders greater physician engagement in network operations. Buy-in is accomplished as part of normal operations rather than separately sought. Trust in the system is enhanced, and the group moves forward more effectively. Of course, all management structures have inherent pros and cons. In the dyad structure, what is gained in alignment and engagement may be offset by a seemingly slower decision-making process and potential ambiguity regarding authority. To foster a successful dyad relationship, you may follow the strategies in exhibit 8.4.

Key Area 4: Keeping Referrals in the Network

During the Strategic Focus phase, referral management or patient referral capture strategy should be addressed. Referral management is an issue that can only be effectively mitigated when a physician–administrator dyad is in place, and this is simply not a reality during the Operational Chaos phase. Some organizations are hesitant to emphasize referral management as a strategy because of existing regulations on directing patients. However, Stark laws and the Anti-Kickback Statute permit internal referrals in an employed physician network as long as exceptions based on patient choice, insurer directives, and provider concerns for quality of care are met. Taking these considerations into account, a network focused on care coordination and consistent best practices will likely deliver superior patient care, creating value and keeping patients in the system.

Drivers of referral leakage
Poor referral capture results from two issues:

1. *Providers directly referring out.* This situation occurs when providers deliberately refer out of network because of

Exhibit 8.4: Fostering Successful Dyad Relationships

Establish the structure. Before filling leadership positions, ensure that the dyad framework is in place. Clearly define the organizational structure, reporting relationships, and expected roles and responsibilities for the dyad pair.

Recruit wisely. A successful pairing begins with the selection process. Selection should consider aspects beyond the requisite job competencies, such as cultural fit with the unit they will lead as well as personality fit with each other.

Set expectations. The pair is expected to work synergistically to execute their well-defined roles and responsibilities. Instill the concept that they are a joint management team who share accountability for the unit's performance and that their roles are complementary rather than duplicative.

Train and mentor the dyad partners. Consider formal and informal education combined with individual and paired coaching to promote a unified function. Left to their own devices, the pair may work separately despite the central structure. If this occurs, dysfunction is the likely outcome.

Educate the network about the dyad's roles and responsibilities, staff reporting relationships, and other issues. Explicitly defining these elements sets realistic, practical expectations. Reliable execution fulfills the expectations and predicts success.

---

previously established relationships, access issues, or quality concerns with in-network physicians and/or resources. This can also occur accidentally when referring providers are confused about who is (or is not) a member of their network. Front-office staff members also contribute to referral leakage; when tasked with making a referral, they take the path of least resistance to securing a referral appointment.

2. *Patients self-referring out.* This situation occurs when a competitor has built a strong brand or market

presence and is able to influence patient perception. Recommendations of friends and family, including those solicited via social media, also play a role. In addition, payers are getting involved in the decision-making process, influencing where patients receive care.

These issues are exacerbated by the lack of a "right-to-win" position for the organization's referral service line, which may result from quality issues with providers and services, not having a full range of care available, problems with timely access, referral roadblocks for referring providers, poor public perception of service offerings, and lack of cost competitiveness.

Develop a referral management strategy

An effective physician network referral management program, with significant engagement by the PAC, has three components:

1. *The right data.* Comprehensive data that detail both employed and independent provider referral patterns are critical to identifying opportunities for improvement. Too often, organizations move forward without data or use incomplete data sets pulled only from their own electronic medical record system, which shows only a portion of the referral pattern picture. Developing a comprehensive baseline of current performance is crucial to uncovering improvement opportunities and building a successful strategy.
2. *A prioritized plan.* Management should prioritize improvement opportunities on the basis of strategic and financial importance. Building an action plan to address right-to-win issues is important as well. No amount of physician engagement will influence providers to refer patients to poor-quality or difficult-to-access services.
3. *Effective engagement and execution.* Many struggling organizations are haphazard in their approach to physician

engagement and outreach. With the right data on hand and a prioritized strategy in place, the dyad management must develop a systematic approach to physician engagement. This approach includes translating strategy into tactics and building the right internal team to execute the plan. Frequently, this appears as a high-functioning physician liaison program that systematically engages providers to prevent issues that cause patient referral leakage.

Organizations with these elements in place enjoy significantly better referral capture outcomes in competitive markets than organizations that are missing one or more of these components.

Key Area 5: Redesigning the Compensation Plan

During the Strategic Focus phase, incorporating incentives that are consistent with network and organizational goals becomes a focus. This means building a compensation plan that rewards not just production but also quality, leadership, team-based performance, and citizenship.

A strategic compensation plan demands providers to be engaged and willing to work with the dyad management to evaluate the correct path forward. To design such a plan, you must have the management infrastructure in place as well as a strategic vision that defines the network's direction. In this way, when future incentives are discussed, providers can gain a clear understanding of why the compensation model needs to evolve. Exhibit 8.5 lists the specific elements of a strategic compensation plan.

Evaluate the compensation structure
Each network's pay plan will ultimately be tailored to its specific situation and market. The following are five recommendations for evaluating a new compensation plan in the Strategic Focus phase:

Exhibit 8.5: Best-Practice Elements of a Strategic Compensation Model

The plan
- receives buy-in and ownership from providers;
- supports a cohesive network culture;
- is consistent with the shared strategic vision;
- contains incentives for productivity levels as well as for quality, patient satisfaction, citizenship, and/or teamwork measures;
- maintains a correlation between individual physician compensation and performance;
- is competitive in the national marketplace but considers unique challenges in the local market;
- is compliant with legal and regulatory requirements;
- is financially sustainable; and
- can be adjusted to shifting revenue streams as the value-based reimbursement model becomes more prevalent.

---

1. *Does it encourage physician leadership?* Clinical skills and knowledge are required to manage and improve quality metrics. Therefore, organizations must engage their best physicians to lead quality improvement programs. However, traditional production-based incentive plans can discourage leadership and involvement in improvement. To leverage your physician talent and support their participation, design a plan that rewards physicians for their leadership, not just their ability to generate work relative value units (wRVUs). Such a plan may offer protected time for administrative duties, prorated wRVU targets, or medical directorships.

2. *Does it incorporate quality metrics?* Incorporating quality metrics in base or bonus compensation will hold physicians accountable for providing high-quality care. Involve them in metric and target selection, which will give them a sense of ownership and present you with meaningful and relevant quality metrics. Start with a

modest pool of quality-based dollars (e.g., $10,000 to $15,000 for primary care) to allow all stakeholders to become comfortable with quality-based payment before significant dollars are at risk.

3. *Is it flexible enough to allow a gradual increase in quality dollars?* Major quality-based payment programs should be phased-in over several years. This ensures that the program has the flexibility to adjust with reimbursement changes and other market factors.

4. *Do the incentives include group pools and/or team goals?* To effect organizational change, physicians and other providers must work together. A properly aligned compensation plan can encourage teamwork and collaboration by focusing on group results or awarding citizenship bonuses to collaborative providers.

5. *Is it structured according to legal parameters?* Those who deal with physician compensation should understand the Stark Law, the Anti-Kickback Statute, and fair market value concepts. By understanding and applying these parameters in the early stages of compensation design, you'll reduce the likelihood of regulatory problems and wasted effort.

Apply the physician compensation structure to advanced practice professionals

Many networks struggle with how to pay advanced practice professionals (APPs). In most cases, the best solution is to mirror the physician contracts, given that APPs are providers and should be contracted for and managed as such. We see many organizations use this formula for their physicians: base + wRVU + quality contracts. However, they pay APPs as nonexempt, hourly employees. This imbalanced pay structure can create misaligned incentives and overall dissatisfaction. Instead, ensure that all providers in the practice are striving toward the same productivity and quality goals. For practices in which the APP bills independently, the APP should be eligible for wRVU-based productivity incentives. For team-based practices, all providers should be held accountable for the combined wRVU target. In all scenarios, APPs should have quality incentives that mirror those of their physician counterparts.

CONCLUSION

The following are the key learning points of this chapter:

1. *Start with a shared vision.* Get physicians involved in developing the network's vision, and make this vision the foundation on which all future priorities and initiatives are built.
2. *Develop a strategic plan.* Strategic planning should be the natural next step after vision creation. If we know where we are going (vision), how are we getting there (strategic plan)?
3. *Expand clinical leadership.* Physician leadership—specifically dyad management—should be in place in the network and should continue as the network grows in size and influence.
4. *Address referral management as a strategic concept.* Referral patterns are slow and painful to change, but avoiding referral problems leads to loss of productivity and sustainability. Get the right data and put them in front of your providers. Then, work with providers to build a referral management strategy within the context of the shared vision.
5. *Evaluate and redesign incentives.* The Strategic Focus phase is the ideal time to reevaluate your compensation strategy to make sure the incentives offered are consistent with your vision and strategic plan.

ADDITIONAL RESOURCE

HSG. 2017. "Physician Network: Building a Shared Vision." http://hsg advisors.com/wp-content/uploads/bsmdw_media/content/Shared_ Vision.pdf.

CASES

The following cases illustrate the concepts discussed in the chapter. The healthcare organizations featured in this section have had a long-term relationship with our consulting practice, HSG, and have given us permission to discuss their employed physician network journey.

St. Luke's Hospital

St. Luke's Hospital in Chesterfield, Missouri, employs more than 110 providers in its medical group and more than 100 in its hospital-based programs. The medical group is an amalgamation of different practices with various specialties and locations. Leadership believed that, for the organization to favorably position itself for value-based care, the medical group had to become more integrated and function as a multispecialty practice.

Approach

A task force of 14 physicians and 3 executives was assembled to define the medical group's vision and the organizational structure needed to support that vision. Interview findings, a self-assessment against best organizational practices, group-specific data analysis, and a St. Louis–region market analysis provided the data that drove the process. A total of four task force meetings were facilitated over a three-month period.

The first meeting focused on defining the process, reviewing the data and interview findings (more than 20 physicians were interviewed along with a half-dozen executives and managers), and discussing the general elements that might be included

continued

in the vision statement. The second meeting focused on presenting local and global industry trends and discussing the potential vision elements in detail. To prompt this discussion, meeting participants were asked to envision the ideal group. What type of group would the physicians be proud of? How would the group need to evolve to meet the market challenges? The third meeting centered on reviewing the initial vision statement draft and the proposed organizational structure. Also discussed was the planned meeting for the entire medical group—a town hall to which all of the employed providers were invited—in which the physicians on the task force would present and solicit physician input on the draft vision statement and the executives on the task force would present the proposed organizational structure. Using task force members for these presentations enhanced physician ownership of the vision process and outcomes.

The fourth and final meeting focused on (1) finalizing the vision statement and organizational structure by incorporating the feedback from the town hall meeting; (2) articulating the culture the physicians wanted to develop and establishing the parameters for that cultural evolution (guided by the results of a detailed survey by task force physicians); and (3) discussing the potential strategic priorities for the medical group, which flowed directly from the vision statement.

Results

The initial implementation efforts focused on physician leadership development. Specifically, St. Luke's selected a chief medical officer for the medical group to work in a dyad relationship with the administrative director. These leaders now jointly chair the Physician Advisory Council (PAC). Along with management, the PAC owns the implementation of the vision. Key elements of this vision are common electronic health record and data analytics systems; a quality plan that tracks across the care continuum and integrates with the inpatient plan; and consistent, positive patient experiences throughout the medical group, regardless of practice or location.

The vision process is a first step in forging a new level of group function and an enhanced partnership between St. Luke's and its employed physicians. This partnership is characterized by physician engagement, mutual accountability, and a joint commitment to the patients.

According to Scott Johnson, vice president and chief financial officer at St. Luke's, "Taking a methodical, inclusive approach to engaging the physicians in the medical group, using an independent consultant, allowed us to work beyond the anticipated challenges of 'management' trying to create a leadership structure for the physicians. HSG was able to help us and our medical group physicians clarify and codify our understanding of our physician culture and the positive relationship administration already has with our physicians, to help us move ahead with a plan for greater physician involvement in medical group leadership. As we establish care coordination infrastructure and engage with our own ACO [accountable care organization] and CIN [clinically integrated network] in the market, a cohesive medical group should make us substantially more responsive and unified in approach."

Hospital System in Northeast Ohio

The employed medical group of a highly successful hospital system in northeast Ohio requested assistance with catalyzing the enhancement of its physician leadership and charting its future course to ensure success in the evolving healthcare

continued

environment. Specifically, the system administration desired to promote a collaborative group function, appropriately enhance the network infrastructure, improve practice operations, cultivate physician leadership, and develop a homogeneous culture and identity. The network experienced significant growth, particularly from 2012 through 2015. Much of the growth occurred through practice acquisition.

The network comprised 146 physicians and 46 advanced practice professionals (APPs) with 19 specialties in 37 locations across 6 counties. The network's management infrastructure did not keep pace and experienced considerable strain. The practices functioned in a semiautonomous fashion: Essentially, they continued much of the operational processes that were in place before their acquisition by the system. Signage initiatives were introduced to create a common identity among the providers, but the network did not have shared culture, operations, or goals.

Approach

In 2015, recognizing the need to effectively communicate with the growing network, the system chartered a committee of physician leaders to enhance bidirectional communication. This committee was not given defined leadership expectations, outside of developing and implementing a communication chain. The network and system leadership presented the network's quality, patient satisfaction, and financial data to the committee, but there was a disconnect between the development of specific action plans and the execution of those plans.

In mid-2016, the system and network leadership undertook a consultative partnership with HSG to catalyze the group maturation process by developing a vision and potential strategies that would best position the network for continued success as the healthcare environment evolves.

To accomplish these objectives, HSG conducted interviews to identify the perceptions about the current status and the future course of the network. Fifteen key physician leaders, the informal nurse practitioner leader, and four key members of the network's administration were interviewed. In addition, select leaders with insight into the network's functionalities completed a formal electronic assessment, measuring the group's functions against 67 targeted best practices, to objectify their perceptions.

Results

To date, the network has accomplished the following:

- Engaged physician leaders in the Leadership Council, turning them into active participants in the group decision-making process
- Added APP representation to the management infrastructure
- Created the following Leadership Council subcommittees: Quality and Patient Experience, Clinical Informatics, and Finance and Operations
- Injected desired physician and APP involvement in operational initiatives, including policy and procedure development and operational standardization
- Addressed several management infrastructure issues
- Enhanced the revenue cycle function, improving the network's patient revenue capture and financial status
- Created the foundation for a cohesive network culture

The network's Leadership Council and administration continue to use the shared vision and associated strategies as a road map for continuing the organization's achievements.

CHAPTER 9

Value Phase

We should seek the greatest value of our action.

—Stephen Hawking

AT THIS POINT in its evolution, the employed physician network is beginning to achieve success in value-based care and one-sided risk contracting. A concerted effort is underway to standardize clinical and operational processes across practice locations, strengthen the shared culture, and define the brand identity. The maturing dyad management and Physician Advisory Council (PAC) are undertaking more complex challenges, such as population health management, compensation plan redesign, risk contracting, clinical practice transformation, and clinically integrated network (CIN) development.

The core characteristics of a network in the Value phase (exhibit 9.1), which overlaps with the Strategic Focus phase, are as follows:

- The network continues to execute its shared vision and associated strategies.
- Providers are now capable of managing to metrics to meet payer requirements and earn financial rewards.
- The maturing dyad management and PAC are pursuing better integration among providers and facing greater challenges.

Exhibit 9.1: Value Phase on the Growth Curve

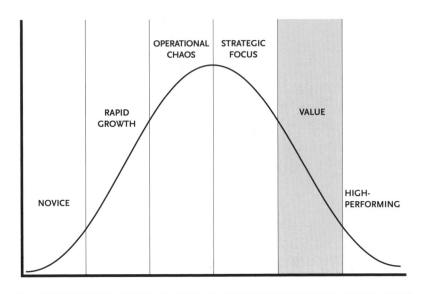

- Refinement and standardization of processes, embedding of a shared culture, and brand identification across practice locations are priorities.

Networks frequently exhibit the characteristics associated with more than one evolutionary phase, but this phenomenon occurs most frequently during the transition from Strategic Focus to Value. Strategies to achieve the shared vision defined during the Strategic Focus phase will mature at different rates and will be implemented at different times throughout the Value phase. As a result, some strategies, programs, or priorities will enter the Value phase sooner than others.

THE EIGHT ELEMENTS IN THE VALUE PHASE

The following is an overview of the eight elements of an employed network in the Value phase:

1. *Strategy.* The Value phase is the period during which strategies from the vision process are launched. Achieving, refining, and expanding these strategies are the network's main activities.

2. *Culture.* Operational standardization, program development, and physician leadership serve as catalysts for the evolution of a shared culture. This shared culture reflects common expectations and behavioral norms and aids with the establishment of a brand identity across the network. The culture supports high physician engagement, which reinforces the focus on clinical best practices.

3. *Quality.* Documented high-quality and cost-efficient care is a hallmark of the Value phase. Likewise, consistently outstanding customer service and experience are institutionalized. Coordination of care across the continuum and proactive patient engagement promote these outcomes. These elements become key characteristics and expectations associated with the network's brand.

4. *Physician leadership.* The designated physician–administrator dyad and the PAC have matured and are driving network progress. During the Value phase, leadership development programs are created to identify and cultivate future leaders among the providers.

5. *Management infrastructure.* Management and technological infrastructures need to evolve during this phase to fully support care coordination, population health management initiatives, clinical integration, risk contracting, and other programs. Increasingly sophisticated data analytics is required to accomplish these objectives.

6. *Aligned compensation.* Incentives that reward more than just productivity are introduced into the pay structure to keep pace with changing organizational strategies and initiatives. Group incentives to promote team-based care and population health management may be implemented.

7. *Brand.* The network brand is starting to be defined and to reflect the emerging culture. Customer expectations become aligned with the brand, and the brand determines customer expectations, regardless of practice location or provider identification.

8. *Financial sustainability.* During the Value phase, financial investments made in previous phases begin to reap rewards in the form of higher patient care revenue, cost avoidance, and cost efficiencies. These results not only allay concerns about the network's financial sustainability but also fuel its growth.

KEY AREAS OF MANAGEMENT FOCUS

Strengthening and implementing the strategies that arose from the shared vision process are the main pursuits in this phase. The key areas of management focus in the Value phase are discussed in this section.

Key Area 1: Mobilizing the Physician Advisory Council

The PAC now plays a key role in network decision making and the resolution of operational issues. As the PAC and its subcommittees mature, they take on more complex responsibilities that directly affect processes and outcomes. Expanding the PAC's role as the central driver for change results in the following:

- Greater physician and advanced practice professional (APP) involvement in initiatives particularly and in network success generally
- Better operational and strategic decisions and performance
- Improved market reputation

The PAC should work with the dyad management in all network activities, including key areas 2 to 8. In addition, it should be empowered to become the catalyst and champion of initiatives, such as improving care coordination among different providers and adopting best practices.

Key Area 2: Adopting a New Compensation Plan

As the network matures, provider compensation plans generally require attention. Most must be redesigned to reward the behaviors and goals necessary to succeed under value-based reimbursement. The incentives themselves must be reformulated because they often focus only on individual production. Individual productivity targets can be antithetical to group functioning and network principles as well as team-based and value-based care delivery. Incentives that reward individual work can lead to micromanagement of practice operations and incite defensive posturing when practice operations are examined, among other consequences. Although individual productivity (or a similar measure of individual effort) will likely remain an essential part of compensation plans, it should not be the sole focus.

Use metrics
Value-based reimbursement offers a plethora of measures or metrics that should be

- customized according to network strategies and vision,
- pertinent to provider specialty,
- reviewed with the providers regularly (e.g., quarterly), and
- revised annually (to ensure the measures are still relevant and represent a true improvement opportunity).

Quality metrics to consider may include measures for accountable care organization (ACO) or Merit-Based Incentive Payment System participation, standards endorsed by specialty societies, and/or clinical practice guidelines. Quality metrics and productivity metrics are not necessarily mutually exclusive. Some networks limit productivity bonuses for physicians who do not meet quality targets, essentially using quality measures as a hurdle. For example, a physician might produce at the 80th percentile but not be compensated at that level unless quality targets are met. The network's compensation plan may cap compensation at the 60th percentile without achievement of quality objectives.

Customer service measures have traditionally been related to patient satisfaction but could be expanded to patient engagement metrics such as the following:

- Number of secured emails initiated or response time to patient emails
- Number or type of appointments scheduled through the patient portal
- Number or type of features publicly accessible through the patient portal (i.e., not private or limited-access content such as test results)

Operational efficiency measures have traditionally focused on meeting budget parameters but could be expanded to other operational areas such as patient access and cost-per-case metrics. Team-based measures should be introduced in the compensation plan to further mitigate the "every man for himself" mentality of individual productivity incentives and to promote group functionality and accomplishments. All of these measures are amenable to group incentive development. For example, a practicewide group productivity incentive allows faster and more effective integration of a new provider or an APP into the practice.

Incorporate APPs into the plan
Inclusion of APPs acknowledges their value and promotes a common direction for all direct care providers. Having a separate, straight-salary compensation structure for APPs aligns neither providers

with each other nor APPs with organizational objectives. The same concept can be applied when incorporating similar individual and group metrics into the performance review process.

Involve the PAC in compensation redesign
Modifying compensation plans can present some key challenges for management. Changing compensation is always a touchy subject for physicians, who often don't view things in the same way as executives do. Direct involvement of the PAC from inception to implementation of the compensation plan can help overcome this challenge. Holding town hall meetings with all providers also gives dyad management an opportunity to explain the revised plan and providers an opportunity to ask questions about it.

Time it right
Keep in mind that a compensation plan redesign is usually more conducive to a steps-based change process than to a sweeping, disruptive process (although it may take longer). With a steps-based approach, it is more likely to garner provider acceptance and support. The timeline of a redesign must parallel the evolution of care delivery models and risk contracting so that the associated incentives make sense. Don't get too far ahead of the reimbursement process. Fee-for-service reimbursement emphasizes face-to-face encounters. Capitated (full risk) reimbursement eschews face-to-face encounters (except when truly necessary) because they are the most expensive care option. Alternative measures in areas such as care management, telehealth, and out-of-office interactions may be required during the transition from fee-for-service to full risk reimbursement.

Make it simple
The new compensation plan should be simple enough to be readily understood and to make an impact. If it is too complex or uses too many metrics, it may be counterproductive and may not produce the desired results.

Key Area 3: Transforming Clinical Practice

Transformation of the clinical care delivery model brings additional capabilities and thus value to practices. It is a next-level venture that relies on adequate infrastructure and a sound operational framework. It is analogous to addressing Maslow's hierarchy of needs: People's basic needs must be fulfilled before they can take on higher levels of function.

Although not required for success, formal programs such as the Centers for Medicare & Medicaid Services (CMS) Transforming Clinical Practice Initiative or the National Committee for Quality Assurance (NCQA) patient-centered care delivery models provide a common, proven set of principles for clinical transformation. Participation in these programs affords a head start and mitigates the effect of internal biases. The framework offered by these programs presents a foundation on which to establish common expectations for all specialties across the network to synergistically promote the shared culture and greater organizational reach. Working toward a common purpose catalyzes the shift from isolated silos to a cohesive collective.

NCQA has programs that are pertinent to most specialties in the network. Patient-centered medical home (PCMH) tenets apply to primary care specialties of family medicine, general internal medicine, and general pediatrics. Patient-centered specialty practice (PCSP) tenets apply to most other specialties. Patient-centered connected care (PCCC) tenets apply to episodic care provided in urgent care centers, retail clinics, and rehabilitation facilities.

These standards outline expectations and outcomes but do not explicitly dictate how practices should meet the standards. They promote team-based care delivery models for all specialty areas but do not delineate or mandate a specific model of care, giving networks the latitude to adopt processes suited to their local circumstances and capabilities. Truly successful participation in formal programs requires eschewing a "checking the box" mentality and focusing instead on pursuing, effecting, and sustaining true change.

Clinical practice transformation can generate additional dividends, such as the following:

- Greater patient, staff, and provider satisfaction and engagement
- Higher-level and more comprehensive care, with increased concentration on preventive services, proactive patient contact, and meaningful data collation
- Better performance on quality metrics
- Lower risk of provider burnout, because patient care responsibilities are spread among a broader care team
- Enhanced attractiveness as a potential partner in a CIN, an ACO, or another value-based initiative

In addition, transformation enables networks to provide value to their patients, practitioners, practice staff, organizations, and other partners.

Pursuing clinical practice transformation presents several key challenges for the dyad management. The first is overcoming inertia. How do you create a sense of urgency to change from the familiar status quo? A shared vision that defines how care will be delivered and will be coordinated can help. It is also important to identify, acknowledge, and address those things that providers and staff are afraid to lose in the process. This is an essential part of change management.

The second challenge is overcoming the impression that the initiative is just about checking a box instead of effecting true change and doing the right things for the right reasons. This challenge is often complicated by preconceived notions that network practitioners have about formal programs or their underlying distrust of initiatives espoused by organizational leadership.

Faced with these challenges, the dyad management must embark on the transformation path with a bit of faith—and maybe outside resources—to overcome the short-term negatives. Chief among those negatives is the short-term financial impact on the organization. The initial investment in clinical transformation will not be offset immediately by increased revenues, and many of the expected returns are either indirect or cost avoidant. The costs associated with implementing and maintaining PCMH programs can be daunting as well. Articulating, emphasizing, and maintaining organizational focus on the anticipated return on investment can overcome short-term misgivings.

Key Area 4: Improving Referral Management

Referral management programs that ensure that appropriate business stays in the network remain a key priority during the Value phase. In the Strategic Focus phase, retaining business is all about generating revenue, but in the Value phase, it is all about care coordination and quality. Keeping the patients under the care of one coordinated team using one coordinated electronic medical record (EMR) helps produce value for the patients.

As noted in chapter 8, determining why referrals leave the system can help networks address important internal issues and improve care delivery. By identifying the gaps in capability, the weakness in quality, and the nonresponsive providers, the dyad management can take the necessary corrective actions. Pursuing PCMH, PCSP, and PCCC recognition across the network can facilitate this process because they underscore the importance of referral relationships.

Key Area 5: Leveraging the Network Brand in the Market

A maturing network that is producing value engenders an identifiable brand that can be leveraged to enhance payer relationships and increase geographic market share. A common approach to demonstrating the ability to produce value is to show quality and cost performance achievements by the organizational employee population. Such data play a central role during contract discussions with commercial insurers and large employers interested in direct contracting.

Entering the payer partnership arena presents some key challenges. First, many networks have no experience contracting with commercial payers or employers. Payer partnerships have traditionally come under the organizational purview, which concentrates negotiations on high-ticket services (e.g., inpatient care, surgery, advanced imaging) rather than on the reimbursement rate for professional services. Although value-based reimbursement is slowly changing this emphasis, it still represents a potentially significant barrier for management to overcome.

Beyond system issues, the network may not have sufficient influence with the insurer to drive, or even steer, the agenda. After all, the insurer is already a primary beneficiary of the network's enhanced performance. The next challenge is convincing the insurer to share the financial rewards it realized through the network's efforts.

Because insurers usually promote varying areas of care, shifting metrics, and different patient populations, proving the network's value to all payers and insurers can be a challenge, even with a tremendously capable network and support structure. Focusing on the priorities for the primary payers in the market only partially overcomes this obstacle, but a network's positive track record with the payer often serves as a solid foundation for unique dialogues about options.

Leveraging the network to broaden its geographic market share is often a progressive process. As the network develops an identifiable brand that reliably provides high-quality care and outstanding customer service, it develops greater recognition in the market. The network becomes an entity that can be effectively marketed and not just advertised. As the brand matures and its reputation spreads, the network becomes the provider of choice. It begins to capture a larger percentage of the primary and secondary service areas and attracts patients from competitors.

Key Area 6: Developing and Expanding Care Management, Care Coordination, and Patient Navigation

Components of clinical practice transformation, care management, care coordination, and patient navigation are initiated during the later stages of the Strategic Focus phase, but they increase in depth, breadth, and sophistication during the Value phase. These programs emphasize the following:

- Risk stratification of the population to target interventions according to individual patient risk
- Incorporating effective disease management systems into the chronic care management program and team-based delivery
- Robust data analytics not adequately provided in the existing EMR

Maturation of these programs is necessary to effectively manage entire populations, which is a hallmark of High-Performing networks.

Key Area 7: Initiating a Population Health Management Program

Population health management is another component of clinical practice transformation. Expanding the breadth, depth, and reach of a population health management program is a cornerstone of progress in the Value phase.

This initiative has its own considerations and complexities. Investment in building or acquiring information systems and data analytics capabilities is required to manage the identified population. These capabilities often extend beyond the standard clinical and practice management informatics systems. Patient registries that interface with electronic systems inside and outside the organization are a necessity, as are access to health information exchanges with unrelated organizations and direct interconnectivity with payer claims databases.

Provider compensation incentives must keep pace with evolving initiatives and programs. Many population health initiatives involve indirect patient care efforts that run counter to the individual productivity incentives common in the fee-for-service environment. Thus, compensation plans need to be modified so that they are not counterproductive.

Key Area 8: Developing or Participating in a Clinically Integrated Network

Throughout the Value phase, many organizations consider parlaying their network into a CIN or participating in a CIN. Clinical integration strategies vary according to regional market forces. CMS encourages CIN development through its ACO offerings, and organizations may contemplate CIN development or participation solely on the basis of this CMS ACO opportunity. However, the true driving force behind most CINs is what's happening in the local market. What are other organizations doing? What pressures are commercial payers exerting?

By definition, CINs actively align and integrate local independent practices with hospitals and health systems to enhance patient care and increase service availability. This advantage can be a significant motivator in many markets, especially if an organization is concerned about encroaching competition or maintaining crucial services in the community but does not want to employ physicians. The principles, best practices, challenges, failures, experiences, lessons learned, achievements, and infrastructures associated with operating and managing a maturing employed physician network are directly applicable to a CIN and can accelerate its success. In addition, independent physicians are much more likely to respect and join an organization that has demonstrated the ability to develop and manage an employed physician enterprise that produces value.

Just fulfilling the legal requirements for a CIN requires a significant investment, regardless of the shared infrastructure with a successful employed network. Joint contracting opportunities are often the impetus to form a CIN, which offsets operating costs and thus motivates independent physician participation. If you plan to pursue risk contracting, enter only those with upside risks (i.e., contracts that use a shared-savings model) and look to gain valuable insights and experience in the process. Only after the CIN has proved its effectiveness in a low-risk environment should you enter contracts with downside risks. Regardless of increasing CMS and congressional pressure, with greater shared-savings potential and guaranteed increases in physician reimbursement (through the Medicare Access and CHIP Reauthorization Act Advanced Alternative Payment Model pathway), you can lose big money if you don't know what you're doing.

CONCLUSION

Following are the key learning points of this chapter:

- During the Value phase, the network builds on, refines, and implements the strategies defined in the shared vision process.
- Standardized practices, a shared culture, and an identifiable brand are some of the characteristics of networks in this phase.
- Clinical practice transformation, designed to facilitate care coordination and population health management, is a key activity.
- The network expands its capabilities to take on increasingly complex issues, such as an evolving compensation plan

with incentives that match the evolving care delivery focus and functions.

- The network begins to demonstrate measurable, rather than theoretical, value; this value engenders an identifiable brand that can be leveraged in the marketplace.

ADDITIONAL RESOURCE

HSG. 2018. "Clinical Practice Transformation." http://hsgadvisors.com/thought-leadership/white-paper/clinical-practice-transformation/.

CASE

The following case illustrates the concepts discussed in the chapter. The healthcare organization featured in this section has had a long-term relationship with our consulting practice, HSG, and has given us permission to discuss its employed physician network journey.

Health System in Kentucky

The employed physician network of St. Claire Healthcare in Morehead, Kentucky, leveraged its capabilities to create a program that drastically reduced the number of patients with chronic pain who received opioid prescriptions. More than 1,000 patients in this program discontinued chronic opioid use, representing greater than 30 percent of the identified network patients with ongoing prescriptions. The network achieved

continued

this quality improvement outcome through collaboration, planning, and strategy implementation.

The network leadership sought opportunities to improve patient outcomes, especially those linked to population health management. The community is in one of the regions with the highest rate of opioid addiction and overdose but with scarce resources available to address the issue. Taking on this kind of performance improvement project would have been inconceivable for the network as recently as two years ago, when it was a disjointed, unfocused medical group that lacked organized physician leadership and a cohesive organizational structure and culture. As system executives considered how to evolve the group into a true multispecialty network that could ultimately manage population health, they explored options to create change and to gain the momentum needed for the network investment to produce value.

Approach

Together, employed network physicians and health system executives developed a 3½-page shared vision document that defined the ideal future group (targeted as ten years hence). It centered on how the network must evolve to meet the needs of the patients, the providers, and the system and to become a group with which physicians would be proud to be associated.

The resulting shared vision consisted of ten primary elements, which became the network's constitution and guide. Three of the vision elements are as follows:

1. Formally designate physician leaders, embedded in a revised organizational structure and supported with a formal Physician Advisory Council, which would enable the network to capture physician insights.

2. Pursue and adopt clinical best practices, particularly those related to population health, and systematically

incorporate them into daily patient management activities.

3.   Value provider well-being, acknowledging that building a great group is not possible if the providers do not feel respected, engaged, and happy with the group.

The newly recruited primary care physician leader faced several issues:

- the desire to identify and implement a performance improvement initiative based on clinical best practices that would produce favorable patient outcomes;
- regional and organizational concerns that opioid use was too high;
- wide variation in physician opioid prescribing without apparent justification for that variation; and
- the daily toll that dealing with "drug seekers" was taking on network providers, who perceived they had no resources to help them effectively deal with the situation.

To address these challenges, the network initiated a population health program using a four-pronged approach:

1.   Document and evaluate the variation in opioid prescribing, and get the physicians to agree that the variation was not justifiable.

2.   Define a standardized process for helping patients with chronic opioid use. The process involved expert medical pain management, an opioid screening clinic staffed by physicians trained in palliative care medicine, and a standard opioid weaning protocol.

continued

3. Develop the resources required to implement the process.
4. Achieve a consensus view that all patients with recurring opioid prescriptions needed to be screened and, if advisable, would enter the weaning protocol.

Program leaders who reviewed the data identified approximately 3,200 network patients with ongoing opioid prescriptions who would be eligible for this initiative. They theorized that at least half of these patients could be weaned from their opioid treatment.

Results

In less than a year from the program's initiation, more than 1,000 patients have successfully discontinued their chronic use of opioids. Patient and physician acceptance of the approach and the resulting outcomes has been high. Physicians are pleased with the perceived improvement in patient care and with the fact that they and their patients are well supported by appropriate resources to combat this significant public health issue.

The program continues to work with the remainder of the original 3,200 patients while monitoring provider adherence to the established prescribing guidelines and recruiting additional participants. The network has also started to plan the next phase of the program: addressing opioid use for acute pain management.

CHAPTER 10

High-Performing Phase

Excellence is never an accident. It is always the result of high intention, sincere effort, and intelligent execution; it represents the wise choice of many alternatives— choice, not change, determines your destiny.

—Aristotle

AN EMPLOYED PHYSICIAN network in the High-Performing phase (exhibit 10.1) is well supported and has mastered the skills and processes that elevate it as an asset—not just as another cost center to the hospital or health system. The network has finally "arrived" as a dominant force in the market and represents the standard to which other networks aspire. However, a High-Performing network cannot rest on its laurels. A continual improvement mentality must be promoted throughout the network to counter the natural force of entropy that erodes the network's advantage. High-Performing networks still face challenges, which are discussed in this chapter.

The core characteristics of a High-Performing network are as follows:

- It expertly enters and manages risk contracts and engages in downside risk.

Exhibit 10.1: High-Performing Phase on the Growth Curve

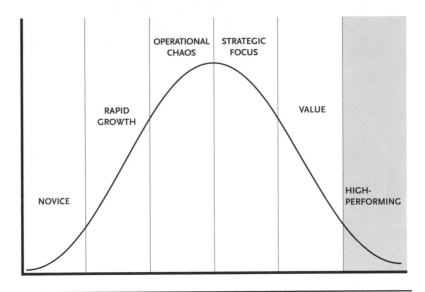

- It continually builds on strengths developed in the Value phase.
- Its growth and operations are stable.
- The capabilities and culture necessary for seamlessly coordinating and managing the health of a defined population are well developed and supported.
- It epitomizes the value equation of delivering cost-effective high-quality care and outstanding patient experiences in a provider-friendly environment.
- It is regarded as the provider of choice, a reputation that is leveraged in the marketplace.

When exactly does a network enter the High-Performing phase? The timing is widely variable, and few networks have reached this level of performance. One main indicator that your network has arrived is that it can successfully manage risk contracts. Being a high performer is often verified through external interactions and assessments, such as payer desires to partner with the network.

THE EIGHT ELEMENTS IN THE HIGH-PERFORMING PHASE

A network in the High-Performing phase handles the eight elements as follows:

1. *Strategy.* Strategy remains central at this point. Much of the strategy relates to reinforcing care management capabilities as well as using information and data to identify and apply best practices. Pursuing strategic growth opportunities is also critical, by leveraging both capabilities and brand equity. Another priority is acquiring or expanding technological and data analytics systems.

2. *Culture.* The well-established culture advances the network's reputation not only in the community and the region but also nationally and even beyond. Recruiting providers who fit the culture becomes easier as candidates approach the network for inclusion. Cultural fit is emphasized, and the culture is clearly exhibited in daily operations. These efforts to sustain the culture, in turn, promote network growth.

3. *Quality.* Consistently good clinical outcomes, outstanding patient experience and engagement, use of updated technology and tools, highly qualified providers, and high patient satisfaction rate are among the indicators of quality. The network also strives to improve the health of its defined population.

4. *Physician leadership.* Leadership development and succession planning become a key focus in the High-Performing phase. As the network's excellent reputation spreads, it attracts more providers and partners, but it can become a victim of its own success as well if it fails to anticipate or plan for staff and leadership attrition. Normal workforce losses through retirements are compounded by attrition that occurs as physicians leave to pursue

career advancement at other organizations or leadership opportunities not available within the network. These losses can pose a threat to leadership sustainability.

5. *Management infrastructure.* High-Performing networks continually reassess their infrastructure to ensure that it is adequate to support the current state and anticipated growth. A specific area of focus is the acquisition of data analytics systems to inform improvement initiatives, financial analytics, and risk contracting.

6. *Aligned compensation.* The compensation plan is regularly reviewed to ensure its alignment with the network's evolving strategic plan, goals, and initiatives.

7. *Brand.* Two brand elements are given special attention in this phase: (1) reputation for reliability with payers and (2) consistent delivery of excellent patient encounters.

8. *Financial sustainability.* The matured, successful network is no longer worried about survival. It can now afford to assume increased contracting risks with bigger payoffs and huge potential losses.

KEY AREAS OF MANAGEMENT FOCUS

Even though process gains have become inculcated in daily operations, energy and accountability must be devoted to maintaining the significant progress to date while continuing to move forward strategically. The key areas for management focus during the High-Performing phase are summarized in this section.

Key Area 1: Maintaining the Organizational Culture

Maintaining the network's culture is a constant challenge, despite the stability of operations, finances, clinical practices, and recruitment strategy. Provider turnover—as a result of personal or family decisions, professional opportunities, and inevitable retirement—needs to be proactively anticipated and addressed so it does not negatively affect the established culture. Although the network's culture is introduced during recruitment and emphasized during onboarding, it requires continued inculcation into new physicians, advanced practice professionals (APPs), and other staff members as they perform daily duties. Perpetuating the culture takes resources, energy, and perseverance.

Key Area 2: Balancing Clinical and Operational Emphases

In High-Performing networks, attaining and maintaining a balance between clinical and operational emphases is the norm, a daily expectation. In previous phases, the focus has been either on administrative or clinical capability, but in this phase, one cannot be favored over the other. Two factors make this balance possible: (1) a dyad management structure that has become synergistic and (2) the Physician Advisory Council and its subcommittees that are involved in driving both aspects. As clinical programs, such as population health management, are established, a blend of operational and clinical considerations must emerge to support those programs. Expansion of these programs increases the number of physician leaders within the network and promotes effective use of operational support services.

Key Area 3: Engaging in Leadership Succession Planning

Succession planning is key to preventing a leadership void. For both physician leaders and administrators, identifying, developing, and involving new leaders is an ongoing commitment. The informal processes used to identify and develop potential future leaders tend to be superseded in this phase by formal programs—whether created internally or pursued externally. Identifying future leaders progresses to incorporating position-specific personality profiles to validate personal impressions. Investment in leadership development shifts from individual pursuit of personal and professional development to organizationally supported internal academies or endorsed external programs. High-Performing networks consider direct investment in future leaders to be critical to their continued success.

Key Area 4: Broadening the Provider Mix Under a Value-Based Environment

The development of complementary provider strategies is important for High-Performing networks in a value-based care environment. Recruitment according to criteria—such as community need, market demographics, and data-driven specialty ratios—has long had advocates. Value-based care tenets and associated team-based care delivery models, however, place new pressures on the provider mix, both by specialty and provider types. Concerns about projected physician shortages accentuate this area's importance.

Developing, expanding, and promoting the full use of a strong primary care base becomes an even greater point of emphasis for value-based care delivery and a lynchpin for population health management. Success in this effort means (1) placing a sufficient number of excellent primary care providers throughout a community to maximize convenient, timely patient access and (2) regarding these providers as a primary source of care, not merely as gatekeepers. To maximize service delivery and provider utilization, all team members must fulfill their duties at the top of their capabilities within licensure constraints. This team-based care model promotes the transition from a system driven by absolute physician numbers to a system driven by relative physician numbers and APPs. It highlights physician-specific skill sets, maximizes patient-centric access and care delivery, and offsets progressive physician shortages (particularly in primary care).

For networks in the High-Performing phase, integration of resources to make the primary care practices the singular source of essential patient services is an ingrained practice. Under this arrangement, behavioral health, care management, and social services can be accessed at the primary care center. Achieving this level of function and accommodating care delivery changes make the traditional benchmark values for metrics, such as staff per provider and square footage per provider, obsolete.

As value-based care programs broaden and become more sophisticated, integrating additional specialty areas becomes another key to success in the High-Performing phase. Developing multispecialty and multidisciplinary programs and centers is a common strategy, because these endeavors are comprehensive, patient-centric, efficient, and cost-effective. Examples of such programs include the following:

- Cardiovascular institutes with cardiologists, cardiothoracic surgeons (location specific), nutritionists and patient educators, and pertinent diagnostic modalities (e.g., stress testing, echocardiography)
- Diabetes centers with endocrinologists, educators, nutritionists, and durable medical equipment (These centers are already replacing stand-alone endocrinology practices, even outside academic environments.)
- Musculoskeletal centers with orthopedists, sports medicine specialists (usually primary care sports medicine physicians), physiatrists, rheumatologists, physical and occupational therapists, orthotics, and basic or advanced imaging capabilities

In addition, High-Performing networks are incorporating more APPs to enhance access and maximize physician reach. Reimbursement models will likely accelerate these changes as initiatives such as bundled-payment initiatives (e.g., the Comprehensive Care for Joint Replacement model) become more common.

Key Area 5: Pursuing Growth Through Market Intelligence

The network, regardless of phase, must remain open to strategic growth opportunities and identify community needs and market opportunities. Community needs change, sometimes abruptly, with changing demographics and market resources. The network must remain flexible to anticipate and meet changing circumstances. Market intelligence is the key to identifying opportunities and avoiding missteps. Active involvement in the community and listening to informal feedback from community members are helpful in collecting market information.

Relationship liaison (or physician liaison) programs are formal programs designed to proactively develop and strengthen the network's professional relationships. The heart of the program is a specially trained individual who understands your business and possesses a personal skill set for cultivating relationships. Usually, such programs focus externally, to enhance referral relationships and develop business opportunities, but liaison activities should go beyond extolling the network's capabilities. They should provide real-time data and information on network strengths, weaknesses, and marketplace changes that offer growth opportunities or could detrimentally affect key services. This information allows the network to consistently meet changing market needs and to remain the provider of choice. See Chay (2015) and Tiller-Hewitt HealthCare Strategies (2018) for more information on designing, implementing, and sustaining a relationship or physician liaison program.

Key Area 6: Achieving Top-Decile Performance

Achieving benchmarked top-decile performance for quality, customer service, and cost are essential to remaining a provider of choice. Comparative benchmarks will progressively rise as more groups dedicate resources for office-based quality program performance, behaving like the hospital-based benchmarks that preceded them.

Opportunities for improvement always exist, and continual performance improvement must remain a hallmark of the network to ensure streamlined processes and desirable outcomes. A provider-of-choice designation depends on top-decile performance in all aspects of network operations and interactions. Demonstrating continued excellence to payers and potential care partners is what ultimately sets High-Performing networks apart.

Key Area 7: Integrating New Data Analytics and Other Information Technology Tools

Proactively managing the health of defined populations and maintaining outcomes at the top decile requires information technology (IT) capabilities not currently available in most electronic health record (EHR) systems. Advanced care management software, disease registries, and data analytics that are integrated into and seamlessly interface with the existing clinical and practice management EHR are all crucial to population health management programs.

In earlier network evolutionary phases, networks often "make do" with workarounds for obtaining the measurement data they need. Significant investments in IT must be balanced with the network's development phase and relevant outcomes. When a network reaches the High-Performing phase, it can afford to upgrade the suboptimal methodologies it tolerated during the early stages. Continued network evolution often mandates additional investments in IT and personnel to permit greater programmatic achievements and more effective outreach. Technology that complements and interfaces with existing platforms and software minimizes interference or disruptions in daily operations. It also enables peak internal functionality and generates relevant information and data, including those that demonstrate network results and capabilities shown to payers and potential care partners.

Key Area 8: Exercising Caution Regarding Partnership Opportunities

High-Performing networks can now contemplate opportunities, such as the following, that were not feasible in earlier phases:

- Creating or being the catalyst of a clinically integrated network (CIN)
- Combining with other CINs to form a super CIN
- Pursuing ambitious risk-contracting opportunities with payers
- Assuming the role of payer through more aggressive direct contracting programs or actual health plan development

Although, at this stage, networks and their parent organizations may begin to feel invincible, they should proceed with caution because endeavors at this level present unique challenges.

CIN strategies are typically driven at the organizational level to steer provider alignment in the market and leverage the network in the process. However, some networks drive the CIN development. As the network becomes accustomed to the CIN's alternative payment models, it may expand the CIN to create the critical mass required for ultimate sustainability and success. Expansion, in turn, may necessitate entering joint ventures with one or several other CINs to form a super CIN. Each level of CIN involvement comes with additional complexities, any or all of which could divert valuable network resources—to the detriment of network functioning and performance.

The basic principle of progressive risk-contracting strategies is to reliably achieve successful performance in an upside-risk-only environment before accepting any downside risk. In partnering with payers, the network may accept financial risk to implement clinical initiatives, such as developing care management capabilities, in exchange for achieving associated performance metrics.

Realizing favorable financial outcomes from clinical practice transformation models may depend on the degree of immersion in risk contracting. A recent study suggested that nearly two-thirds of reimbursement contracts may need to be based on capitation (full risk) to sustain clinical practice transformation (LaPointe 2017).

CONCLUSION

Although the High-Performing network has fully matured, it must actively seek opportunities to continually improve and evolve; otherwise, it risks complacency and stagnation. The following are the key learning points of this chapter:

1. Leadership succession planning, provider development, and managing physician attrition are critical to achieving and maintaining high levels of performance.
2. Complementary IT and analytics systems are necessary to advance network capabilities and overcome previously tolerated but suboptimal solutions.
3. The established culture must be inculcated in daily operations and among new hires.
4. Ultimately, the network's reputation is defined by its clinical outcomes, patient experience and engagement, and access to services.
5. Broadening the provider mix to deliver the best results will grow in importance.
6. Partnerships and relationships can leverage the capabilities of the network, but a cautious approach must be taken.

REFERENCES

Chay, A. 2015. "Implementing a Physician Liaison Program." Physicians Practice. Published January 14. www.physicianspractice.com/partnerships/implementing-physician-liaison-program.

LaPointe, J. 2017. "63% Capitation Needed to Sustain Primary Care Transformation." *RevCycle Intelligence*. Published September 6. https://revcycleintelligence.com/news/63-capitation-needed-to-sustain-primary-care-transformation.

Tiller-Hewitt HealthCare Strategies. 2018. "How a Physician Liaison Delivers a Competitive Advantage." Accessed August 13. www.tillerhewitt.com/wp-content/uploads/2018/08/How-a-Physician-Liaison-Delivers-A-Competitive-Advantage.pdf.

PART III

Additional Concerns and Conclusion

CHAPTERS 11 TO 13 address two critical issues:

1. The employed physician network's interactions with independent physicians in the community, and how to engage them in a mutually beneficial way
2. The development of relevant metrics and dashboards, and how these tools need to evolve along with the network

The last chapter highlights the multilayered value that networks add to the hospital or health system, and it reinforces the lessons from this book. Of all the endeavors healthcare organizations are pursuing today, an employed physician network is the one that offers the best opportunity to improve patient care in communities.

We hope that this book spurs you to think about your current environment and, most important, to act on moving forward on your employed physician network journey.

CHAPTER 11

Alignment and Integration with Independent Practices

Alliances and partnerships produce stability when they reflect realities and interests.

—Stephen Kinzer

PHYSICIAN ALIGNMENT AND integration are keys to success in a value-based care environment. Thus far, we have focused on one part of physician alignment and integration—the employed physicians. However, hospitals and health systems cannot afford to lose sight of the other part—independent physicians with private practices, who are becoming a minority presence in the community as a growing percentage of medical staffs enter employed relationships.

Physicians may prefer to remain independent for various reasons, such as the desire to maintain full autonomy or the perception of unthreatened practice sustainability. These independent practices need to be actively engaged to get all local physicians (and medical staff members) pulling in the same direction and achieving mutually beneficial outcomes for the physicians, the organization, and their shared patients. Although physician alignment has always been important, it is pivotal in the value-based reimbursement era. The crucial role of alignment became readily apparent during the early hospital-based pay-for-performance initiatives involving patient experience (Hospital Consumer Assessment of Healthcare Providers and Systems reporting), quality of care (core measures and avoidable hospital-acquired conditions), and utilization (length of stay and readmission rates).

Organizational and physician reimbursement models are becoming increasingly intertwined with initiatives such as bundled payments. These initiatives affect not only payments and incentives but also reputation (as results are publicly reported).

PHYSICIAN PARTICIPATION IN STRATEGIC PLANNING AND IMPLEMENTATION

Health system strategic planning is a high-profile endeavor in which both independent and employed physicians should be intimately involved. Direct input from the beginning to the end of the process is indispensable to both long- and short-term success, especially if broad physician representation is pursued. With such input, plan implementation tends to be better received, and physicians are more likely to remain active throughout the plan monitoring and review processes. Without such input, physicians tend to lose interest. Participation by both independent and employed physicians in these processes promotes the open sharing of viewpoints, which creates a mutual understanding between these "competitors." Failure to engage physicians leads to responses that range from total apathy to total defiance and suboptimal performance.

Regardless of the tactics deployed, the organization should show respect for the entire physician community and be proactive and transparent in communicating with independent physicians to earn their trust. Ask for their recommendations about the most effective means to communicate with physicians, and then ask them to champion the communication plan among their peers. Sharing information about work groups acting on their behalf, initiatives being considered, and progress being made goes a long way toward generating physician involvement with the organization and with each other.

SHARED PERSPECTIVE OF NETWORK AND INDEPENDENT PHYSICIANS

The network must maintain and enhance its relationship with independent practices in the service area. Both parties should work together to develop a mutually beneficial agreement, created from their shared perspective and expectations. This process may lead to a synergistic relationship rather than friction or animosity.

To initiate this conversation, the parties can focus on the patient referral process, discussing reciprocal expectations about referring and consulting specialties. Many networks have developed formal expectations in this area, and those expectations often became the basis of relationships with private physicians. The National Committee for Quality Assurance Patient-Centered Medical Home and Patient-Centered Specialty Practice standards can also serve as a foundation for gaining a mutual understanding of each other and their respective patient care approaches.

Forging any kind of a professional relationship requires a proactive, transparent approach. Avoid mystique and intrigue. Share information about changes in strategic direction or new initiatives, keeping in mind that independent practices also forward the organization's vision by meeting the community's needs. The better informed the independent practices are, the more aligned they can be and the more willing they are to promote mutual success.

Creating a formal relationship liaison program at the network or organizational level can help avoid awkwardness. The relationship liaison should be viewed as a bidirectional communication vehicle as opposed to a unidirectional sales force. Complaints from independent practices should be welcomed and addressed, and their input should lead to process improvement and enhanced services. A robust relationship liaison program not only builds greater alignment through enhanced, open relationships but also provides opportunities for internal review based on external input. Learning how private practitioners perceive the network providers is valuable.

ALIGNMENT AND INTEGRATION MECHANISMS

Various mechanisms can be used to promote alignment and integration of independent physicians, including both formal legal structures and informal arrangements.

Healthcare organizations can develop formal alliances that legally permit closer, mutually beneficial relationships with independent physicians in their communities. These legal structures must conform to applicable legislative and regulatory requirements to ensure that collusion does not occur or is not perceived to have occurred. An early example of this formal legal structure is the physician–hospital organization (PHO) and its variations. In the 1990s, PHOs enabled organizations to become full-service providers to managed care payers and employers. For physician members, PHOs offered greater reimbursement opportunities.

Clinically Integrated Networks

Spurred by the Medicare Shared Savings Program and guided by the US Federal Trade Commission, clinically integrated networks (CINs) represent a significant opportunity to partner with independent community physicians to achieve the Triple (or Quadruple) Aim: higher quality of care at a lower cost with greater patient satisfaction and engagement (while considering or enhancing physician well-being).

All CINs must be designed to enhance quality of care throughout the integrated network. This aim is accomplished through the use of standardized metrics and the implementation of proven clinical practice guidelines and best practices. In addition, the mandated governance structure requires broad provider inclusiveness, shared direction, and progressive improvements in outcomes. The organization, employed physicians, and independent physicians in a CIN immediately share a common interest, which promotes close cooperation and collaboration.

CINs present a real opportunity for elevating interrelationships, patient outcomes, and mutual financial benefits, but pitfalls can still occur. For example, the CIN may not achieve a shared savings payout. Members may become disillusioned when the CIN fails to attain the quality performance metric or to meet financial performance goals. Worse, if the CIN enters a contract with downside financial risk and incurs a penalty, physician members can be adversely affected. The financial risk must be delineated for all involved. In addition, CIN membership requires physicians' active participation. They must not only be aware of the quality reporting requirements but also strive to improve metric performance, actively follow clinical practice guidelines, and enhance the care collectively provided in the CIN. Although these expectations are included in CIN participation agreements, clearly defining them during initial discussions with potential physician members prevents surprises later and lays the foundation for a transparent, trusting relationship.

Joint Ventures

Joint ventures are formal legal partnerships between an organization and independent physicians to undertake a specific purpose. They tend to be somewhat limited in scope and relate to a specific venture, such as an ambulatory surgery center, a stand-alone imaging center, or a medical office building. These arrangements may closely align the participants involved, but they primarily form for financial reasons—to increase revenue or to minimize revenue loss.

Despite being limited in scope, joint ventures are fraught with risks and can strain relationships between partners. Issues of governance and management control are common, and the parties may have perspectives that are diametrically opposite. A venture's less-than-desired financial performance may cause conflict, and underperformance is a real possibility in an environment of declining reimbursement rates. If the venture is profitable, the strain may come from parties that feel alienated or left out and that demand their financial status and viability be elevated in some fashion. In addition, a joint venture may put at risk an organization's nonprofit designation. Joint venture development entails satisfying significant, complicated legal and regulatory requirements, of which prospective physician partners may be unaware. A not-for-profit organization must be cognizant of the potential effects of the venture.

Given its limited scope and potential risks, joint ventures seem to be falling out of favor, especially with the rise of CINs, which address a multitude of needs in a value-based care environment.

Formal Leadership Roles

The formal service line or departmental medical director position provides a mechanism for incorporating independent physicians in network or organizational operations. Such a position requires a professional services agreement with many stipulations.

Another mechanism is an appointment to serve on an organizational-level Physician Advisory Council. This group consists of organizational executives, independent physician leaders, network dyad management, employed physicians, and potentially board members who discuss current market trends, strategic and operational challenges, recruitment and retention of new physicians in the community, and other issues. This type of council has a proven track record of spurring better working relationships between the members and leveraging those relationships to stimulate the creation of physician-driven initiatives, especially those related to quality of care, patient experience, cost-effectiveness, and value-based care delivery. This approach can help define realistic expectations for all parties and encourage aligned actions and behaviors.

Administration should be extremely cautious about overtly inter-loping in medical staff functions, but opportunities to encourage independent physician involvement in roles such as department chairs, medical staff officers, or at-large medical executive committee members can be worthwhile. This mechanism can minimize percep-tions that the organization is interested in the employed network only, and it ensures the independent physician voice is present and heard.

Comanagement Agreements

Comanagement agreements can be mutually beneficial for the orga-nization and the involved physicians. They target improvements in quality of care and patient satisfaction, as well as reductions in operating costs, by offering pay and incentives to participating phy-sicians. These agreements answer the query, "What's in it for me?" when independent physicians are asked to actively and aggressively work on issues that seem to primarily benefit the organization.

Most comanagement agreements are formal and include base fees for hours dedicated to comanagement activities, such as attending project meetings, and incentive fees for achievement of predefined quality metrics in targeted areas. The combination of payments is designed to motivate physicians to achieve the desired behaviors and outcomes.

A comanagement agreement must clearly delineate duties the physicians must perform to be eligible for both base and incentive payments. Base-fee duties often include the following:

- Participation in multidisciplinary performance improvement meetings
- Development of standardized treatment protocols and care guidelines
- Resource planning and technology development, including equipment or device standardization

- Education for other providers, nurses, and staff members
- Contribution to strategy and marketing

For the incentive fee, the agreement delineates performance metrics and targets relevant to quality of care, patient safety, patient satisfaction, and operational efficiency. The incentives vary by circumstance and year, must represent true opportunities to reach a stretch goal, and must be reevaluated and updated regularly (often annually).

Metric and target selection, which should be agreed on by all parties, is one of the most challenging aspects of implementing a comanagement agreement. Proper selection of metrics and targets is not only crucial to achieving success but also ensures that the agreement meets fair market value (FMV) and commercial reasonableness requirements to avoid Stark Law and Anti-Kickback Statute issues. Using national measures and benchmarks allows the objective evaluation of service line performance. Reliance on standardized data raises the agreement's credibility among physicians, streamlines data collection and reporting, and facilitates regulatory and statutory compliance.

In addition, comanagement agreements can be used to address call-coverage issues. More and more physicians are requesting payment for emergency department and inpatient call coverage, and organizations want to avoid setting that precedent. Thus, including a call-coverage requirement as a prerequisite for participation in the comanagement agreement can prevent conflict and misunderstanding. Many organizations have proverbially "killed two birds with one stone" in this fashion. See exhibit 11.1 for a checklist of specific tasks related to comanagement agreement development.

Professional Services Agreements

A professional services agreement (PSA) generally involves contracting for local services from a large regional practice, health system, or academic center. However, at times, a PSA can be used with local practices to address service gaps, such as by improving the

Exhibit 11.1: Comanagement Agreement Checklist

_____ Understand the basics of comanagement.

_____ Complete a baseline assessment of service line performance.

_____ Identify potential metrics for the incentive fee.

_____ Focus the assessment on quality metrics that have a defined financial effect and/or metrics established by professional organizations.

_____ With physicians, finalize metrics and select targets.

_____ Define tiers of accomplishment if applicable (for example, what level gets 60%, 80%, or 100% payout?).

_____ Establish duties payable at an hourly rate.

_____ Define a cap on the number of payable hours.

_____ Determine the fair market value hourly rate.

_____ Determine the fair market value of the incentive payments.

_____ Establish a payout schedule.

_____ With attorneys, define the breakdown of the compensation opportunity for hourly work versus incentives.

_____ With attorneys, review compliance and fair market value issues.

_____ Draft legal contracts.

_____ Establish meeting schedules.

_____ Ensure physicians have appropriate resources.

_____ Monitor metrics/performance.

_____ Monitor physician hours.

---

availability of a specialist for consults or providing geographic coverage in a new market. One example might involve the need for an outpatient pulmonologist for two half-days per week, located and supported in space leased from the hosting institution. Another example might involve efforts to make professional services available to satisfy requirements for a formal designation, such as a designated trauma center or primary stroke center. In this scenario, designation might require a provider to have on-call availability for a low-demand specialty (such as ophthalmology coverage in a designated trauma center). Each of these examples calls for a PSA that details the specific services and the mutual expectations of the involved parties.

The most straightforward PSA pays the service provider for a specific time or services commitment at a specialty-specific FMV rate; for example, four hours of schedulable patient care time two days per week at a rate of $XX per hour (FMV rate for specialty). The PSA also stipulates that the host organization will bill and retain the professional service reimbursements to offset the provider costs. Travel time and indirect care time (e.g., encounter documentation) should be clarified. Clearly delineating the desired service arrangement helps manage expectations, prevent misunderstandings, and minimize withdrawal of services.

PSAs are often used to compensate physicians in formal leadership positions, such as medical staff officers, department chairs, and clinical service line medical directors. These arrangements require clearly delineated performance expectations and compensation, calculated according to an FMV administrative reimbursement rate (not specialty-specific unless required by a position like clinical department chair). They also must stipulate the timely submission of compliance documentation (actual hours spent per listed duty) before payment is given (often monthly or quarterly).

PSAs can be used to transition an independent practice to an employed practice when an incumbent provider prefers to remain independent. This scenario occurs when a provider is retiring soon and planning to "surrender" the practice to the organization after the retirement date. Rather than wait for the date, the organization acquires and begins to manage the practice ahead of time. The practice staff members who stay on become employees of the organization, and the provider is retained at an FMV rate through the retirement date. In this way, the organization can begin the recruitment, selection, and even onboarding processes of the replacement physician ahead of schedule, allowing for a smooth transition. More important, this arrangement ensures the continuity of services in the community while allowing the provider to remain independent. The provider legally retains independent status insofar as she is not employed, but she has relinquished full autonomy because the practice has been acquired by the organization. This relationship must be clearly defined and well understood during the negotiating process.

Management Services Organizations

The traditional management services organization (MSO) was a formal legal structure in which the organization or its employed provider network provided defined practice management services to independent practitioners. Practices could select from a menu of services that were designed to alleviate administrative burdens, such as revenue cycle management (billing), human resources support for staffing, and full management of the practice.

The traditional MSO model was based on several interrelated principles:

- The organization or network had greater resources and expertise to perform administrative or business functions.
- The practices wanted to focus on clinical care and considered administrative functions a burden on their limited time.
- Outsourcing practice management was mutually beneficial (e.g., it allowed for economies of scale).
- The arrangement promoted organization–physician alignment.

In theory, the MSO was an attractive physician alignment mechanism for the organization. In practice, however, it presented significant performance risks. The organization had to deliver a product or service that met or exceeded the practice's expectations, which were unrealistic at times. Failure to meet these expectations risked straining the relationship. Over time, the MSO began to lose favor—whether because the organization could no longer justify the risks or it wanted to engage in outright employment or acquisition.

Today, a new version of the MSO model is emerging in some markets, as independent practices approach organizations for assistance with value-based care initiatives. The new MSO services include clinical informatics and data analytics support, performance improvement expertise, Medicare Access and CHIP Reauthorization Act (or MACRA) participation guidance and assistance, and care management or population health resources. One underlying principle of the traditional MSO remains: The practice wants to remain independent but cannot find a practical path to meet various regulatory or advanced care delivery requirements. This option may be critical for organizations that cannot—or do not want to—accommodate every practice that requests employment but desires to assist and maintain alignment with local independent practices.

Many elements of the new MSO model are central to CIN operations. This model helps position the organization and practices for future CIN development by aligning the practices with organizational processes and addressing immediate value-based care needs.

CONCLUSION

Alignment and integration of independent physicians are gaining even greater importance as the transition to value-based care progresses. Most organizations and networks cannot fully achieve success without independent physicians. Many mechanisms exist to promote alignment and integration. Organizations should select the mechanisms that permit customized approaches to meet organizational and community needs. The long-term sustainability of organizations and networks will depend on their ability to forge an effective, mutually beneficial relationship with independent physicians.

ADDITIONAL RESOURCES

Articles

Ansel, T. 2015. "Physician Alignment Strategy … Solving the Puzzle, Part One." HSG. http://hsgadvisors.com/thought-leadership/articles/physician-alignment-strategy-solving-puzzle/.

Barker, N. 2015. "Physician Alignment … Solving the Puzzle, Part 2." HSG. http://hsgadvisors.com/thought-leadership/articles/physician-alignment-solving-puzzle-part2/.

CASE

The following case illustrates the concepts discussed in the chapter. The healthcare organization featured in this section has had a long-term relationship with our consulting practice, HSG, and has given us permission to discuss its employed physician network journey.

Hospital System in the Mid-Atlantic Region

A two-hospital system was experiencing inefficiencies in its catheterization laboratory, resulting in high costs per case, substandard outcomes, and diminished market share. The lab was used by interventionalists from two different independent cardiology groups. With HSG, the system administration explored several alignment methods, including employment, call-coverage pay, and professional services agreements. Ultimately, a comanagement agreement was selected as a viable and cost-effective solution.

Approach
Baseline assessment was performed by comparing cost, satisfaction, and quality data with national benchmarks. On the

continued

basis of these results, a list of draft metrics was compiled, and the interventional cardiologists selected five metrics to be included in the comanagement agreement. A list was generated to specify the duties for which the physicians would be paid under the contract, including education and training sessions with emergency department and cath lab staff members, as well as local emergency medical services units.

Results
- Both the interventional cardiologists and system administration were pleased with the comanagement agreement and dedicated efforts to improve performance:
  - The system allotted resources to more reliably and effectively collect and report data to a recognized national registry.
  - The interventional cardiologists invested time and energy to improve their performance against the metric targets. In the first year, they exceeded three out of the four quality goals.
- The comanagement agreement has been renewed annually since its inception five years ago and was recently introduced to different independent groups practicing at a second site.
- The accomplishments to date are as follows:
  - The group now meets or exceeds all but two national registry benchmarks, compared with zero when the comanagement agreement was initiated. An example is door-to-balloon time decreasing from an average of 90 minutes at baseline to 59 minutes.
  - The average cost per case in the cath lab was reduced from $2,309 to $1,303 (a 44 percent absolute decrease) before the addition of an

intervention to decrease site-compression requirements.
- The interventional cardiologists adopted a proactive approach to improving care delivery:
  - They significantly increased use of the radial approach over the femoral approach (rarely used at baseline but now the preferred approach for appropriate patients).
  - They introduced an intervention that decreases the incidence of femoral insertion site bleeding (incidence decreased to zero for the most recent 12-month interval from a baseline of 3.3 percent and previous nadir of 0.61 percent); reduces the length of time nurses have to apply direct compression of the site; and decreases patient observation time.
- Each performance improvement initiative has increased unit efficiency and improved patient outcomes.
- Enhanced performance has translated to improved reputation in the community and increased market share compared with the direct competition.

The comanagement agreement has led to significant engagement of the independent interventional cardiologists, improved cath lab operations, and enhanced patient outcomes—all of which have elevated the system's reputation in the market. Everyone involved in this comanagement agreement views it favorably. The system has already engaged another set of interventional cardiologists at a second cath lab location and may approach other specialties (e.g., orthopedics) in a similar fashion.

CHAPTER 12

Dashboards as a Network Management Tool

What's measured improves.

—Peter F. Drucker

DASHBOARDS ARE VISUAL, graphical, or numerical summaries of performance in all or any areas or programs that the hospital, health system, or employed physician network wants to measure, monitor, and manage. They serve four key purposes. First, they create a system for management control. Second, they enable leaders to manage risks. Dashboards organize multilayered data to make them understandable or easier to follow. With this information, leaders in High-Performing networks can better anticipate and prepare for risks and thus make decisions about entering risk contracts. Third, dashboards promote a culture of accountability because progress (or lack of progress) is tracked and displayed. In many ways, this is the most important use of dashboards, particularly in new businesses such as employed physician networks. But as many healthcare executives know, building a culture of accountability among physicians is a complex task. Fourth, dashboards serve as an excellent board education tool. They illustrate to board members the network's objectives and the metrics for those objectives. We recommend routinely sharing a subset of the executive dashboard with your board.

An *executive dashboard* is the macro view of overall performance, indicating what strategic objectives are being met, being exceeded, are on track, are falling behind, or need immediate intervention. An *operational dashboard* is the micro view of performance at the unit level—for a network, this is the specialty or practice—indicating achievements or inadequacies in specific measures or metrics, programs, activities, and so on. In this way, both executives and managers can pinpoint problem areas and systematically resolve them before they spiral out of control. This chapter focuses on the executive dashboard, although the operational dashboard is briefly discussed.

AREAS OF FOCUS

Dashboards need to be organization specific. The areas or categories that executives need to monitor and control vary on the basis of organizational needs, the management team's capabilities, and market specifics. In general, dashboards should include metrics in five areas:

1. *Quality.* The dashboard should include both outcomes and process measures, but more outcomes measures should be added as the network matures. Compliance with national standards mandated by the Centers for Medicare and Medicaid Services (CMS) or other payers should take a prominent position, and many quality measures will be based on the network's quality plan. The network may perform better on measures that are of interest to the practices rather than those forced on them by outside entities. Pertinent metrics will reflect the network's phase of maturation. During the clinical transformation process, one metric that might be considered is the percentage of practices certified as a patient-centered medical home or a patient-centered specialty practice (if the network has embarked on this path). As the group undertakes risk contracting, performance on quality hurdles—objectives

that must be achieved before financial incentives can be paid out—becomes important.

2. *Patient experience and access.* Ease of access at the practice level is an essential operational measure to track, regardless of the network's maturity. Measures of the third appointment available is a good access metric; it is better than next-available appointment, which is subject to more random variation. Measures of patient satisfaction with the practice and the provider are also important. Clinician and Group Consumer Assessment of Healthcare Providers and Systems (CG-CAHPS) metrics for the overall provider composite measure is a good starting point.

3. *Volume and throughput.* This category may overlap with the patient experience and access measures. For the executive dashboard, include productivity measures such as work relative value units (wRVUs) per provider and productivity percentile based on benchmarks. Specialty capture rate is another good metric because it indicates leakage from the network, but note that not all referral leakage is the same. For example, out-of-network referrals to loyal physicians should be measured differently from referrals to competitors. Likewise, referral to resources not available in the network should be recognized as appropriate.

4. *Revenue cycle.* Given the challenges in the Operational Chaos phase (challenges often associated with revenue cycle failures), the revenue cycle metrics shine a light on poor performance. Report revenue cycle metrics separately from other financial measures. Our preferred metrics are as follows:
   - Days in accounts receivable
   - Adjusted collection rates, which measure performance against maximum potential collections (the best overall measure of revenue cycle performance)
   - Total professional collections
   - Collections per wRVU versus benchmark

5. *Operations.* Some organizations need metrics as basic as physician and advanced practice professional full-time equivalents (FTEs). Major financial outcomes are good as well and should include the following:
   - Net income or loss
   - Net income or loss per provider
   - Overhead rate
   - Provider cost as a percentage of revenue
   - Correlation between productivity and compensation (Our preferred latter measure is variation on a scatter diagram, and the percentage of physicians compensated 10 percent from the norm on the basis of productivity.)

As the network enters risk contracts, some measure of financial performance under those contracts is required as well.

EXECUTIVE-LEVEL VERSUS PRACTICE MANAGEMENT–LEVEL INFORMATION

In working with clients, we often see confusion over how much information is appropriate for inclusion in dashboards. The most frequent mistake is including the same level of data in the executive dashboard (distributed to organizational executives) as in the operational dashboard (distributed to practice managers). This distinction gets lost at times, causing the executive to miss the forest for the trees. The system's chief financial officer, for example, should not receive dashboards that contain too much detail because this leader's main concern is the overall financial health (the forest), not specific expenses, revenue, and other finance-related numbers (the trees). A short explanation of the operational dashboard is in order here before we move on to our main discussion of the executive dashboard.

Operational dashboards contain essential data on practice priorities and are designed for use by practice managers or practice administrators. They provide feedback and guidance to those most invested in the practice's functions—physicians and other staff. Among the day-to-day operational details included are health insurance claims denials, FTE costs, and subsets of the CG-CAHPS. The metrics shown in exhibit 12.1 illustrate how practice performance contributes to the overall network performance (as illustrated in the executive dashboard).

EXECUTIVE-LEVEL DASHBOARDS: EVOLVING METRICS

Like the networks themselves, dashboards and the metrics used must evolve. At the Novice phase of the growth curve, the number of providers may be tracked. At the High-Performing phase of the growth curve, performance on risk contracts may be measured.

In this section, we discuss sample or prototype dashboards containing our recommended metrics for each phase of the growth curve. Exhibit 12.2 outlines all of the metrics, and the subsequent exhibits show the metrics that may be added to or deleted from the dashboard as the network matures and grows in size. In the exhibits, metrics that are essential to each phase are bolded, and optional metrics are light gray.

In the Novice phase, network management should limit the number of basic measures included on the dashboard. Limits are recommended for two reasons. First, the management infrastructure at this point is not robust and likely has limited ability to collect the data. Second, management should focus on metrics that can help the network avoid future problems. Issues such as overpaying physicians or tolerating low productivity levels need to be monitored and managed early. Mastering the revenue cycle is likewise critical. In the first three phases (from Novice to Operational Chaos), patient experience and quality metrics are generally managed at the practice level (using operational dashboards), because the managerial infrastructure is either nonexistent or still developing and thus cannot appropriately address problems that arise. We recommend using six metrics during the Novice phase (exhibit 12.3).

Exhibit 12.1: Sample Operational Dashboard

Metric	Current Year YTD if Appropriate	Prior Year	Variance vs. Prior Year	Goal	Variance vs. Goal
Quality/Patient Experience					
CG-CAHPS (Access to Care Top-Box Score)	60%	50%	10%	90%	–30%
CG-CAHPS (Provider Communication Top-Box Score)	80%	70%	10%	90%	–10%
CG-CAHPS (Test Results Top-Box Score)	85%	75%	10%	90%	–5%
CG-CAHPS (Office Staff Top-Box Score)	65%	50%	15%	90%	–25%
MIPS (Quality Measure) *Select a Measure*	75%	70%	5%	80%	–5%
MIPS (Improvement Activity) *Select a Measure*	80%	75%	5%	80%	0%
MIPS (Advancing Care Information) *Select a Measure*	65%	70%	–5%	80%	–15%
Operations					
Total Support Staff FTEs	360	350	10	N/A	N/A
Total Support Staff FTEs per Provider	4.50	6.36	–1.86	3.30	1.20

Total Support Staff FTEs per 10,000 wRVUs	10.29	14.00	−3.71	6.53	3.76
Total Support Staff Cost as a % of Revenue	35.00%	40.00%	−5.00%	28.62%	6.38%
General Admin. Staff per FTE Provider	0.10	0.20	−0.10	0.22	−0.12
Revenue Cycle					
% of AR over 90 Days	35%	55%	−20%	25%	10%
Registration Error Rate	15%	20%	−5%	7%	8%
Claim Denial Rate	11%	15%	−4%	7%	4%
Late (Delinquent) Charges Rate	6%	10%	−4%	5%	1%
Point-of-Service Collection Rate	73%	60%	13%	90%	−17%
Volume/Throughput					
Avg. Time to Third Available Appointment (in Days)	12.00	14.00	−2.00	7.00	5.00
% of Appointment Slots Filled per Day	74%	65%	9%	95%	−21%
No-Show/Same-Day Cancellation Rate	15%	25%	−10%	8%	7%

Note: AR = accounts receivable; CG-CAHPS = Clinician and Group Consumer Assessment of Healthcare Providers and Systems; FTE = full-time equivalent; MIPS = Merit-Based Incentive Payment System; wRVU = work relative value unit; YTD = year to date.

Exhibit 12.2: Dashboard Metrics for Evolving Networks

Metric	Current Year YTD if Appropriate	Prior Year	Variance vs. Prior Year	Goal	Variance vs. Goal
Quality					
Quality Improvement Initiative #1	49	40	9	60	–11
Quality Improvement Initiative #2	49	40	9	60	–11
Quality Improvement Initiative #3	49	40	9	60	–11
% Certified PCMH/PCSP	61%	42%	19%	80%	–19%
Patient Experience/Access					
CG-CAHPS (Overall Provider Rating Composite)	70%	80%	–10%	90%	–20%
Days Until Third Appointment (Average by Practice)	5.6	10.4	4.8	3	–2.6
Operations					
Physician FTEs	50	35	15	61	–11
APP FTEs	30	20	10	32	–2
Net Income or (Loss)	($20,000,000)	($13,750,000)	($6,250,000)	($17,300,000)	($2,700,000)
Net Income or (Loss) per Provider	($250,000)	($275,000)	$25,000	($240,000)	($10,000)
Overhead Rate (Operating Expenses as % of Revenue)	50%	60%	–10%	45%	5%

Metric					
Total Provider Cost as % of Revenue	60%	70%	−10%	60%	0%
Provider Comp vs. Productivity (% Outside 10% Corridor)	25%	30%	−5%	10%	15%
Medical Loss Ratio/Performance on Risk Contracts	96%	102%	6%	89%	−7%
Revenue Cycle					
Days in AR	45.0	60.0	−15	35	10
Adjusted Collection Rate	90%	85%	5%	99%	−9%
Professional Collections per wRVU	$100	$100	$0	$120	($20)
Volume/Throughput					
wRVUs Total (Personally Performed Only)	350,000	250,000	100,000	370,000	−20,000
wRVUs per Provider (Personally Performed Only)	4,375	4,545	(170)	4,982	(607)
Referral Capture Rate	80%	60%	20%	90%	−10%

Note: APP = advanced practice professional; AR = accounts receivable; CG-CAHPS = Clinician and Group Consumer Assessment of Healthcare Providers and Systems; FTE = full-time equivalent; PCMH = patient-centered medical home; PCSP = patient-centered specialty practice; wRVU = work relative value unit; YTD = year to date.

Exhibit 12.3: Metrics for the Novice Phase

Metric	Current Year YTD if Appropriate	Prior Year	Variance vs. Prior Year	Goal	Variance vs. Goal
Quality					
Quality Improvement Initiative #1	49	40	9	60	–11
Quality Improvement Initiative #2	49	40	9	60	–11
Quality Improvement Initiative #3	49	40	9	60	–11
% Certified PCMH/PCSP	61%	42%	19%	80%	–19%
Patient Experience/Access					
CG-CAHPS (Overall Provider Rating Composite)	70%	80%	–10%	90%	–20%
Days Until Third Appointment (Average by Practice)	5.6	10.4	4.8	3	–2.6
Operations					
Physician FTEs	50	35	15	61	–11
APP FTEs	30	20	10	32	–2
Net Income or (Loss)	($20,000,000)	($13,750,000)	($6,250,000)	($17,300,000)	($2,700,000)
Net Income or (Loss) per Provider	($250,000)	($275,000)	$25,000	($240,000)	($10,000)
Overhead Rate (Operating Expenses as % of Revenue)	50%	60%	–10%	45%	5%

Total Provider Cost as % of Revenue	60%	70%	-10%	60%	0%
Provider Comp vs. Productivity (% Outside 10% Corridor)	**25%**	**30%**	**-5%**	**10%**	**15%**
Medical Loss Ratio/Performance on Risk Contracts	96%	102%	6%	89%	-7%
Revenue Cycle					
Days in AR	**45.0**	**60.0**	**-15**	**35**	**10**
Adjusted Collection Rate	90%	85%	5%	99%	-9%
Professional Collections per wRVU	$100	$100	$0	$120	($20)
Volume/Throughput					
wRVUs Total (Personally Performed Only)	350,000	250,000	100,000	370,000	-20,000
wRVUs per Provider (Personally Performed Only)	4,375	4,545	(170)	4,982	(607)
Referral Capture Rate	80%	60%	20%	90%	-10%

Note: APP = advanced practice professional; AR = accounts receivable; CG-CAHPS = Clinician and Group Consumer Assessment of Healthcare Providers and Systems; FTE = full-time equivalent; PCMH = patient-centered medical home; PCSP = patient-centered specialty practice; wRVU = work relative value unit; YTD = year to date.

In the Rapid Growth phase, the financial risks grow as more providers join the network. At this point, we recommend a number of other financial metrics, such as provider cost as a percentage of revenue. However, without a dyad management system, physician leadership, or Physician Advisory Council in place, adequately managing quality or referral capture metrics at the network level is rarely possible; such metrics are not added until the Strategic Focus phase. During the Rapid Growth phase, acquiring and onboarding providers are the main focus. Seven metrics may be included on the executive dashboard during this phase (exhibit 12.4).

In the Operational Chaos phase, losses become a burning issue. Increasing the number of providers is no longer the preoccupation, although in some networks the imperative to grow primary care remains critical. In this phase, the network is driven by raising revenue, so access measures receive greater attention, as do all aspects of financial performance. As shown in exhibit 12.5, we recommend including 11 specific metrics on the dashboard for monitoring and managing.

During the Strategic Focus phase, the network begins to view quality as an essential component to realizing the network's shared strategic vision and associated strategic plan. Referral capture as well as patient experience and access are among the areas that are monitored. Ten metrics (exhibit 12.6) are appropriate to include on the executive dashboard for measurement and management.

The exhibit 12.7 dashboard represents the priorities in the Value phase. The network is focused on providing value-based care and achieving the desired value-based outcomes, and in the process, earning incentives from CMS and private insurers. In this environment, multiple quality metrics are monitored. The executive dashboard includes ten metrics that require management focus. As the network gets better control of finances, fewer financial metrics need to be monitored and the focus shifts to summary metrics.

The executive dashboard in the High-Performing phase (exhibit 12.8) looks radically different from the dashboard in the Novice phase. Medical loss ratios (performance on risk contracts), referral capture, and quality metrics dominate. For High-Performing networks, patient experience, access, and satisfaction measures are crucial, and financial metrics have become high-level summary items. To reiterate an earlier point, the network dashboard must change with the objectives of the organization. By definition, a High-Performing network's objectives relate to its ability to achieve predictable outcomes in the areas of quality, cost, and access.

These dashboard examples contain suggested metrics for each phase of the network's evolution. Although you may use the same or similar categories and metrics, you must customize them to fit your network's particular vision, plans, market, and culture.

CONCLUSION

In this chapter, we address several key principles for developing dashboards. We want to emphasize three of these principles in particular:

1. Many hospitals fall into the trap of tracking and reporting too many metrics on the executive dashboard. A lot of excruciating detail could be reported, but executives cannot or do not absorb most of this information. Therefore, the number of metrics must be kept to a manageable number—generally fewer than a dozen at any one time.
2. Higher-level, summary metrics are most valuable to executives who are overseeing an employed network for the first time. Those metrics generally incorporate a number of key processes in the network but serve as an early warning that something is wrong.
3. Metrics need to evolve with the network. Although we explore just the evolution of the group itself, we believe that organizational executives also evolve. Over time, as executives gain knowledge and confidence in their understanding of the network, the metrics of interest will change accordingly.

We hope these recommendations accelerate your progress, challenge your thinking, and guide your development of metrics to help you measure, monitor, and manage your network's performance.

Exhibit 12.4: Metrics for the Rapid Growth Phase

Metric	Current Year YTD if Appropriate	Prior Year	Variance vs. Prior Year	Goal	Variance vs. Goal
Quality					
Quality Improvement Initiative #1	49	40	9	60	–11
Quality Improvement Initiative #2	49	40	9	60	–11
Quality Improvement Initiative #3	49	40	9	60	–11
% Certified PCMH/PCSP	61%	42%	19%	80%	–19%
Patient Experience/Access					
CG-CAHPS (Overall Provider Rating Composite)	70%	80%	–10%	90%	–20%
Days Until Third Appointment (Average by Practice)	5.6	10.4	4.8	3	–2.6
Operations					
Physician FTEs	50	35	15	61	–11
APP FTEs	30	20	10	32	–2
Net Income or (Loss)	($20,000,000)	($13,750,000)	($6,250,000)	($17,300,000)	($2,700,000)
Net Income or (Loss) per Provider	($250,000)	($275,000)	$25,000	($240,000)	($10,000)
Overhead Rate (Operating Expenses as % of Revenue)	50%	60%	–10%	45%	5%

Total Provider Cost as % of Revenue	60%	70%	−10%	60%	0%
Provider Comp vs. Productivity (% Outside 10% Corridor)	25%	30%	−5%	10%	15%
Medical Loss Ratio/Performance on Risk Contracts	96%	102%	6%	89%	−7%
Revenue Cycle					
Days in AR	**45.0**	**60.0**	**−15**	**35**	**10**
Adjusted Collection Rate	90%	85%	5%	99%	−9%
Professional Collections per wRVU	$100	$100	$0	$120	($20)
Volume/Throughput					
wRVUs Total (Personally Performed Only)	350,000	250,000	100,000	370,000	−20,000
wRVUs per Provider (Personally Performed Only)	4,375	4,545	(170)	4,982	(607)
Referral Capture Rate	80%	60%	20%	90%	−10%

Note: APP = advanced practice professional; AR = accounts receivable; CG-CAHPS = Clinician and Group Consumer Assessment of Healthcare Providers and Systems; FTE = full-time equivalent; PCMH = patient-centered medical home; PCSP = patient-centered specialty practice; wRVU = work relative value unit; YTD = year to date.

Exhibit 12.5: Metrics for the Operational Chaos Phase

Metric	Current Year YTD if Appropriate	Prior Year	Variance vs. Prior Year	Goal	Variance vs. Goal
Quality					
Quality Improvement Initiative #1	49	40	9	60	–11
Quality Improvement Initiative #2	49	40	9	60	–11
Quality Improvement Initiative #3	49	40	9	60	–11
% Certified PCMH/PCSP	61%	42%	19%	80%	–19%
Patient Experience/Access					
CG-CAHPS (Overall Provider Rating Composite)	70%	80%	–10%	90%	–20%
Days Until Third Appointment (Average by Practice)	**5.6**	**10.4**	**4.8**	**3**	**–2.6**
Operations					
Physician FTEs	50	35	15	61	–11
APP FTEs	30	20	10	32	–2
Net Income or (Loss)	**($20,000,000)**	**($13,750,000)**	**($6,250,000)**	**($17,300,000)**	**($2,700,000)**
Net Income or (Loss) per Provider	($250,000)	($275,000)	$25,000	($240,000)	($10,000)
Overhead Rate (Operating Expenses as % of Revenue)	50%	60%	–10%	45%	5%

Total Provider Cost as % of Revenue	60%	70%	–10%	60%	0%
Provider Comp vs. Productivity (% Outside 10% Corridor)	25%	30%	–5%	10%	15%
Medical Loss Ratio/Performance on Risk Contracts	96%	102%	6%	89%	–7%
Revenue Cycle					
Days in AR	45.0	60.0	–15	35	10
Adjusted Collection Rate	90%	85%	5%	99%	–9%
Professional Collections per wRVU	$100	$100	$0	$120	($20)
Volume/Throughput					
wRVUs Total (Personally Performed Only)	350,000	250,000	100,000	370,000	–20,000
wRVUs per Provider (Personally Performed Only)	4,375	4,545	(170)	4,982	(607)
Referral Capture Rate	80%	60%	20%	90%	–10%

Note: APP = advanced practice professional; AR = accounts receivable; CG-CAHPS = Clinician and Group Consumer Assessment of Healthcare Providers and Systems; FTE = full-time equivalent; PCMH = patient-centered medical home; PCSP = patient-centered specialty practice; wRVU = work relative value unit; YTD = year to date.

Chapter 12: Dashboards as a Network Management Tool   213

Exhibit 12.6: Metrics for the Strategic Focus Phase

Metric	Current Year YTD if Appropriate	Prior Year	Variance vs. Prior Year	Goal	Variance vs. Goal
Quality					
Quality Improvement Initiative #1	**49**	**40**	**9**	**60**	**–11**
Quality Improvement Initiative #2	**49**	**40**	**9**	**60**	**–11**
Quality Improvement Initiative #3	49	40	9	60	–11
% Certified PCMH/PCSP	61%	42%	19%	80%	–19%
Patient Experience/Access					
CG-CAHPS (Overall Provider Rating Composite)	**70%**	**80%**	**–10%**	**90%**	**–20%**
Days Until Third Appointment (Average by Practice)	**5.6**	**10.4**	**4.8**	**3**	**–2.6**
Operations					
Physician FTEs	50	35	15	61	–11
APP FTEs	30	20	10	32	–2
Net Income or (Loss)	**($20,000,000)**	**($13,750,000)**	**($6,250,000)**	**($17,300,000)**	**($2,700,000)**
Net Income or (Loss) per Provider	**($250,000)**	**($275,000)**	**$25,000**	**($240,000)**	**($10,000)**
Overhead Rate (Operating Expenses as % of Revenue)	50%	60%	–10%	45%	5%

Total Provider Cost as % of Revenue	60%	70%	–10%	60%	0%
Provider Comp vs. Productivity (% Outside 10% Corridor)	**25%**	**30%**	**–5%**	**10%**	**15%**
Medical Loss Ratio/Performance on Risk Contracts	96%	102%	6%	89%	–7%
Revenue Cycle					
Days in AR	**45.0**	**60.0**	**–15**	**35**	**10**
Adjusted Collection Rate	**90%**	**85%**	**5%**	**99%**	**–9%**
Professional Collections per wRVU	$100	$100	$0	$120	($20)
Volume/Throughput					
wRVUs Total (Personally Performed Only)	350,000	250,000	100,000	370,000	–20,000
wRVUs per Provider (Personally Performed Only)	4,375	4,545	(170)	4,982	(607)
Referral Capture Rate	**80%**	**60%**	**20%**	**90%**	**–10%**

Note: APP = advanced practice professional; AR = accounts receivable; CG-CAHPS = Clinician and Group Consumer Assessment of Healthcare Providers and Systems; FTE = full-time equivalent; PCMH = patient-centered medical home; PCSP = patient-centered specialty practice; wRVU = work relative value unit; YTD = year to date.

Exhibit 12.7: Metrics for the Value Phase

Metric	Current Year YTD if Appropriate	Prior Year	Variance vs. Prior Year	Goal	Variance vs. Goal
Quality					
Quality Improvement Initiative #1	49	40	9	60	–11
Quality Improvement Initiative #2	49	40	9	60	–11
Quality Improvement Initiative #3	49	40	9	60	–11
% Certified PCMH/PCSP	61%	42%	19%	80%	–19%
Patient Experience/Access					
CG-CAHPS (Overall Provider Rating Composite)	70%	80%	–10%	90%	–20%
Days Until Third Appointment (Average by Practice)	5.6	10.4	4.8	3	–2.6
Operations					
Physician FTEs	50	35	15	61	–11
APP FTEs	30	20	10	32	–2
Net Income or (Loss)	**($20,000,000)**	**($13,750,000)**	**($6,250,000)**	**($17,300,000)**	**($2,700,000)**
Net Income or (Loss) per Provider	($250,000)	($275,000)	$25,000	($240,000)	($10,000)
Overhead Rate (Operating Expenses as % of Revenue)	50%	60%	–10%	45%	5%

Measure					
Total Provider Cost as % of Revenue	60%	70%	−10%	60%	0%
Provider Comp vs. Productivity (% Outside 10% Corridor)	**25%**	**30%**	**−5%**	**10%**	**15%**
Medical Loss Ratio/Performance on Risk Contracts	96%	102%	6%	89%	−7%
Revenue Cycle					
Days in AR	**45.0**	**60.0**	**−15**	**35**	**10**
Adjusted Collection Rate	90%	85%	5%	99%	−9%
Professional Collections per wRVU	$100	$100	$0	$120	($20)
Volume/Throughput					
wRVUs Total (Personally Performed Only)	350,000	250,000	100,000	370,000	−20,000
wRVUs per Provider (Personally Performed Only)	4,375	4,545	(170)	4,982	(607)
Referral Capture Rate	**80%**	**60%**	**20%**	**90%**	**−10%**

Note: APP = advanced practice professional; AR = accounts receivable; CG-CAHPS = Clinician and Group Consumer Assessment of Healthcare Providers and Systems; FTE = full-time equivalent; PCMH = patient-centered medical home; PCSP = patient-centered specialty practice; wRVU = work relative value unit; YTD = year to date.

Exhibit 12.8: Metrics for the High-Performing Phase

Metric	Current Year YTD if Appropriate	Prior Year	Variance vs. Prior Year	Goal	Variance vs. Goal
Quality					
Quality Improvement Initiative #1	49	40	9	60	–11
Quality Improvement Initiative #2	49	40	9	60	–11
Quality Improvement Initiative #3	49	40	9	60	–11
% Certified PCMH/PCSP	61%	42%	19%	80%	–19%
Patient Experience/Access					
CG-CAHPS (Overall Provider Rating Composite)	70%	80%	–10%	90%	–20%
Days Until Third Appointment (Average by Practice)	5.6	10.4	4.8	3	–2.6
Operations					
Physician FTEs	50	35	15	61	–11
APP FTEs	30	20	10	32	–2
Net Income or (Loss)	**($20,000,000)**	**($13,750,000)**	**($6,250,000)**	**($17,300,000)**	**($2,700,000)**
Net Income or (Loss) per Provider	($250,000)	($275,000)	$25,000	($240,000)	($10,000)
Overhead Rate (Operating Expenses as % of Revenue)	50%	60%	–10%	45%	5%

Total Provider Cost as % of Revenue	60%	70%	−10%	60%	0%
Provider Comp vs. Productivity (% Outside 10% Corridor)	25%	30%	−5%	10%	15%
Medical Loss Ratio/Performance on Risk Contracts	**96%**	**102%**	**6%**	**89%**	**−7%**
Revenue Cycle					
Days in AR	**45.0**	**60.0**	**−15**	**35**	**10**
Adjusted Collection Rate	90%	85%	5%	99%	−9%
Professional Collections per wRVU	$100	$100	$0	$120	($20)
Volume/Throughput					
wRVUs Total (Personally Performed Only)	350,000	250,000	100,000	370,000	−20,000
wRVUs per Provider (Personally Performed Only)	4,375	4,545	(170)	4,982	(607)
Referral Capture Rate	**80%**	**60%**	**20%**	**90%**	**−10%**

Note: APP = advanced practice professional; AR = accounts receivable; CG-CAHPS = Clinician and Group Consumer Assessment of Healthcare Providers and Systems; FTE = full-time equivalent; PCMH = patient-centered medical home; PCSP = patient-centered specialty practice; wRVU = work relative value unit; YTD = year to date.

CHAPTER 13

A Call to Action

Don't manage—lead change before you have to.

—Jack Welch

THE EMPLOYED PHYSICIAN network is an amazing strategic asset. You can grow it to include needed specialties. You can work with the physicians to grow its geographic footprint. You can get a better handle on referral leakage, and you can work with the physicians to ensure that your hospital or health system earns their business. The network can also be an asset with employers, as its capabilities accrue to employers and patients in the community.

Building and nourishing the network may be your best opportunity to improve quality of care in your community. No other program or initiative unambiguously allows the organization to align with physicians and to create an environment in which their mutual goals can be met. In an industry fraught with numerous limits and frustrations, the network offers a great reason for optimism.

VALUE IN EACH EVOLUTIONARY PHASE

The value that the network can produce for a healthcare organization is enormous. In the Novice phase, the network offers physicians the opportunity to preserve or continue their practices in a welcoming employed environment. By inviting physicians to join, the network not only increases patient volume for the organization but also ensures access to basic and specialized healthcare services for the community. These same benefits are replicated in the Rapid Growth phase, when the network's capabilities expand to include more physicians in different specialties.

In the Operational Chaos phase, the network invests in technological systems, managerial infrastructure, and other operational capabilities. These investments strengthen the network and set the stage for better clinical quality, more seamless coordination among providers, and greater community health benefits. Because of financial losses, network management may also begin to focus on referral leakage. This focus not only pays immediate volume dividends but also leads to a more tightly integrated network with better care coordination. As the physicians learn to work as a team and standards are established, variations in clinical care and administrative operations are slowly reduced.

By the Strategic Focus phase, moving a common vision and strategy forward is the norm. The network first produces value by increasing volume in the fee-for-service environment. As the physicians become fully engaged, they become partners who help guide the organization on the path toward value-based care. Patients benefit as the network focuses on improving performance to meet or exceed quality measures.

The network's momentum continues in the Value phase. By this point, the network is managing to the metrics and positively affecting reimbursement by reducing readmissions and hospital-acquired conditions and meeting core measures. The network may leverage these gains by partnering with employers and insurers, which creates a new value equation.

A High-Performing network is a strategic asset. It is adept at managing and coordinating care for a defined population, enabling the organization to benefit from risk contracting. At the same time, it ensures appropriate volume to benefit from fee-for-service arrangements. Knowledgeable physicians provide valuable insights and help with the transition between the two markets.

ASSESSING THE NETWORK'S MOVE FORWARD

What do you plan to do to move forward to the next phase of network evolution? How are you going to build a shared vision, strategic objectives, and dashboards? How are you going to create the organizational accountability required for progress? Addressing these questions (and many others) will get you thinking about the next steps of the employed physician network journey. Ultimately, that may be the main value of this book.

Clear, Shared Vision

- What must this network become to deliver our desired results in the future?
- How do we build a network with which physicians are happy to associate and of which they are proud?
- How do we create a network that delivers value to payers and to the healthcare organization?

Strong Managerial and Technology Infrastructure

- How can we assemble a network management team with the capabilities necessary for success?
- Where do we find the talent, and how do we develop that talent?
- How do we engage physicians and gain their insights?
- How do we acquire the information technology and data analytics systems to guide the network in producing predictable costs and quality?

- What infrastructure can be shared with the organization, and what must be freestanding?

Physician Leaders

What physician leadership capabilities must be built to get to the High-Performing phase?

- How are physician leaders selected? Groomed? Developed?
- How are their roles defined?
- How can we initiate and foster a dyad relationship?

Current Performance

- Do we understand current performance versus benchmarks?
- What type of analysis do we conduct to improve financial performance?
- What changes do we make to realize these improvements?

Growth

- How will the network grow in the future?
- What geographic areas would add value?
- What physician specialties are required to enable more effective care management?
- What additions to the network would solidify the organization's market position?
- What specialties and practices will help reduce referral leakage?

Risk Contracting

- How do we gain a better understanding of what it takes to succeed at risk contracting?
- Should the organization pursue direct contracts with employers?
- Should the organization pursue one-sided risk via the Medicare Shared Savings Program?
- When do we want to be prepared to take full risk?
- How may the network help educate the organization about risk-contracting challenges?

Clinical Transformation Plan

- How do we begin to change the way care is delivered?
- How do we explore and experiment with new care models?
- How do we educate and engage providers to ease the transformation?
- How do we build systems that will produce reliable outcomes and predictable costs?
- How do we build a system, beyond physician practices and hospitals, that provides a continuum of healthcare services?

Plan of Action

- How do we translate our goals into a plan of action?
- How does our vision help us define our priorities?
- How does the vision help us articulate annual objectives and define dashboard metrics?

We encourage you to use the insights, tactics, recommendations, and resources in this book in designing your plan of action.

CONCLUSION

From your current situation, building a network may seem impossible. It will be a long process, up to 10 or 15 years in many cases. The frustrations, setbacks, conflicts, pushback, and financial losses will be daunting at times. Despite all of this, always remember that the journey is about serving patients in the community well, and your organization's best hope for doing so is the High-Performing employed physician network. No other strategic initiative can make a bigger impact on your organization's long-term success.

Thank you for reading this book. Our hope is that, in time, your employed physicians and patients will thank you as well.

Appendix:
HSG Physician Network
Evaluation Survey

THIS SELF-ASSESSMENT SURVEY gauges the employed physician network performance in eight major categories. It should take approximately 10 to 15 minutes to complete. Your honest assessment is critical to the network evaluation's success. Thank you for completing HSG's network evaluation survey.

ROLE SELECTION

Please select your role in the organization.

- ❏ Physician—primary care
- ❏ Physician—specialty care
- ❏ Advanced practice professional (NP, PA, CNS, etc.)—primary care
- ❏ Advanced practice professional (NP, PA, CNS, etc.)—specialty care
- ❏ Hospital administration
- ❏ Practice management/administration
- ❏ Board of directors
- ❏ Other (please specify)

STRATEGY

Our administrative team and physicians have a shared vision of how our network will evolve over time to be a strategic asset for the health system.

- ❑ Strongly disagree
- ❑ Somewhat disagree
- ❑ Neutral
- ❑ Somewhat agree
- ❑ Strongly agree
- ❑ Don't know

Comments: _____

_____

We have a strategic plan for the employed physician network that is used by management and providers to guide decision making within the organization.

- ❑ Strongly disagree
- ❑ Somewhat disagree
- ❑ Neutral
- ❑ Somewhat agree
- ❑ Strongly agree
- ❑ Don't know

Comments: _____

_____

We have the providers and capabilities we need to execute the network's strategy and serve the needs of the health system and community.

- ❑ Strongly disagree
- ❑ Somewhat disagree
- ❑ Neutral
- ❑ Somewhat agree
- ❑ Strongly agree
- ❑ Don't know

Comments: _____

_____

When we identify a provider recruitment need, we are able to effectively recruit and fill that position on a timely basis with a quality provider.

❑ Strongly disagree
❑ Somewhat disagree
❑ Neutral
❑ Somewhat agree
❑ Strongly agree
❑ Don't know

Comments: _____

_____

CULTURE

Our employed physician group has a definable, cohesive culture that is pervasive throughout the group and guides management, provider, and staff behavior.

❑ Strongly disagree
❑ Somewhat disagree
❑ Neutral
❑ Somewhat agree
❑ Strongly agree
❑ Don't know

Comments: _____

_____

We have a clear and standardized process for onboarding newly recruited physicians that reflects and instills the group's culture.

❑ Strongly disagree
❑ Somewhat disagree
❑ Neutral
❑ Somewhat agree
❑ Strongly agree
❑ Don't know

Comments: _____

_____

PHYSICIAN LEADERSHIP

The composition of our physician advisory council is appropriate and has direct input into the network's operations and strategy.

- ❑ Strongly disagree
- ❑ Somewhat disagree
- ❑ Neutral
- ❑ Somewhat agree
- ❑ Strongly agree
- ❑ Don't know

Comments: _____

_____

There is appropriate communication to the provider group, as a whole, about management and physician leadership council activities and decision making.

- ❑ Strongly disagree
- ❑ Somewhat disagree
- ❑ Neutral
- ❑ Somewhat agree
- ❑ Strongly agree
- ❑ Don't know

Comments: _____

_____

MANAGEMENT INFRASTRUCTURE

Our network management team has the depth, resources, and capabilities it needs to successfully operate the network.

- ❑ Strongly disagree
- ❑ Somewhat disagree
- ❑ Neutral
- ❑ Somewhat agree
- ❑ Strongly agree
- ❑ Don't know

Comments: _____

_____

Our IT infrastructure provides the network administrative team the reports and data it requires to effectively and efficiently manage the practices, as well as support value-based initiatives.

- ❏ Strongly disagree
- ❏ Somewhat disagree
- ❏ Neutral
- ❏ Somewhat agree
- ❏ Strongly agree
- ❏ Don't know

Comments: _____

_____

We have an effective management dashboard that measures and tracks key practice and network performance indicators and helps management identify priority issues to tackle.

- ❏ Strongly disagree
- ❏ Somewhat disagree
- ❏ Neutral
- ❏ Somewhat agree
- ❏ Strongly agree
- ❏ Don't know

Comments: _____

_____

Our practices have standardized clinical operations across the network.

- ❏ Strongly disagree
- ❏ Somewhat disagree
- ❏ Neutral
- ❏ Somewhat agree
- ❏ Strongly agree
- ❏ Don't know

Comments: _____

_____

FINANCIAL SUSTAINABILITY

The subsidies required by the network are sustainable at their current rate.

- ❑ Strongly disagree
- ❑ Somewhat disagree
- ❑ Neutral
- ❑ Somewhat agree
- ❑ Strongly agree
- ❑ Don't know

Comments: _____

_____

Our billing function is appropriately set up and staffed to be an effective revenue cycle engine for the network.

- ❑ Strongly disagree
- ❑ Somewhat disagree
- ❑ Neutral
- ❑ Somewhat agree
- ❑ Strongly agree
- ❑ Don't know

Comments: _____

_____

We have an effective administrative process for onboarding new providers and practices, resulting in minimal disruption to practice patterns and revenue cycle.

- ❑ Strongly disagree
- ❑ Somewhat disagree
- ❑ Neutral
- ❑ Somewhat agree
- ❑ Strongly agree
- ❑ Don't know

Comments: _____

_____

Our providers are as efficient and productive as we need them to be for sustainable operation of the network.

❑ Strongly disagree
❑ Somewhat disagree
❑ Neutral
❑ Somewhat agree
❑ Strongly agree
❑ Don't know

Comments: _____

_____

Our network has minimal leakage (in-network provider referrals to out-of-network providers and facilities) for patients that our health system would like to retain.

❑ Strongly disagree
❑ Somewhat disagree
❑ Neutral
❑ Somewhat agree
❑ Strongly agree
❑ Don't know

Comments: _____

_____

QUALITY

We perform well on outcome-based quality metrics.

❑ Strongly disagree
❑ Somewhat disagree
❑ Neutral
❑ Somewhat agree
❑ Strongly agree
❑ Don't know

Comments: _____

_____

Our practices are actively involved in an office-based quality program that is directly linked into the hospital's/system's program.

❑ Strongly disagree
❑ Somewhat disagree
❑ Neutral
❑ Somewhat agree
❑ Strongly agree
❑ Don't know

Comments: _____

_____

Our practices fully embrace team-based care using support staff at the top of their capabilities.

❑ Strongly disagree
❑ Somewhat disagree
❑ Neutral
❑ Somewhat agree
❑ Strongly agree
❑ Don't know

Comments: _____

_____

We have defined standards for "patient access" within the network and succeed at meeting those standards.

❑ Strongly disagree
❑ Somewhat disagree
❑ Neutral
❑ Somewhat agree
❑ Strongly agree
❑ Don't know

Comments: _____

_____

Our network can measure and prove that it delivers great customer service and high patient satisfaction.

- ❏ Strongly disagree
- ❏ Somewhat disagree
- ❏ Neutral
- ❏ Somewhat agree
- ❏ Strongly agree
- ❏ Don't know

Comments: _____

_____

BRAND/IDENTITY

Our employed physician network has an identifiable brand that has been thoughtfully established.

- ❏ Strongly disagree
- ❏ Somewhat disagree
- ❏ Neutral
- ❏ Somewhat agree
- ❏ Strongly agree
- ❏ Don't know

Comments: _____

_____

We are the provider of choice in our market.

- ❏ Strongly disagree
- ❏ Somewhat disagree
- ❏ Neutral
- ❏ Somewhat agree
- ❏ Strongly agree
- ❏ Don't know

Comments: _____

_____

ALIGNED COMPENSATION

Our current provider compensation methodology provides the correct incentives to create alignment with hospital/health system objectives.

- ❏ Strongly disagree
- ❏ Somewhat disagree
- ❏ Neutral
- ❏ Somewhat agree
- ❏ Strongly agree
- ❏ Don't know

Comments: _____

_____

Total provider compensation is regularly reviewed and measured against predefined criteria, such as external benchmarks. Specific criteria determine when external reviews are conducted.

- ❏ Strongly disagree
- ❏ Somewhat disagree
- ❏ Neutral
- ❏ Somewhat agree
- ❏ Strongly agree
- ❏ Don't know

Comments: _____

_____

OVERALL

Please choose the best overall description of your employed provider network, from the statements below:

❑ Our network is dabbling in employment, mainly as a reactive measure, with no growth strategy. Our network lacks a formal management infrastructure and can best be described as a small group of independent physicians who share the same tax ID number.

❑ Our network is beginning to aggregate in size, with some proactive physician employment based on perceptions of strategic need. Our network remains loosely organized and does not have much in terms of dedicated management structure.

❑ Our network has grown rapidly and is now experiencing operational challenges as a result of that growth. Our network is experiencing increasing practice subsidies that must be addressed. Hospital leadership is sensing the need to control the group's growth and limit employment offers to manage the losses of the group.

❑ Our network's growth is mature and operations are relatively under control. Our largest focus is getting providers engaged and building a shared vision and culture, as well as getting providers more involved in leadership and management of the network.

❑ Our network has moved past being concerned with growth, operations, and culture development, and it is largely focused on developing the capabilities needed to provide value to the organization—quality care delivery, care management capabilities, population health, and so on.

❑ Our network is stable in all aspects of management and has developed both the culture and capability to manage populations and take on risk.

Please provide the following contact information to receive your survey results:

Name _____

Company _____

Email address _____

Index

Note: Italicized page locators refer to figures or tables in exhibits.

239

Benchmarks: current performance *vs.*, in employed physician networks, 224; service line performance and, 188; top-decile performance and, 174–75

Billing: in Novice phase, 111; in Operational Chaos phase, 111–12; options for Novice networks, 70; physician acquisitions and, *86*; in Rapid Growth phase, 92, 111. *See also* Central billing office

Board members: dashboards and, 197; educating, in Novice phase, 74–75

Boards, informal, PACs and, 113

Bonus compensation: quality metrics in, 140

Brand: in High-Performing employed networks, 48–49; in High-Performing phase, 56, *59*, 170; in HSG Physician Network Evaluation Survey, 235; leveraging in the market, in Value phase, 158–59; in Novice phase, 55, *59*, 67; in Operational Chaos phase, 55, 56, *59*; in Rapid Growth phase, 55, *59*, 84; in Strategic Focus phase, 55, 56, *59*, *130*; in Value phase, 56, *59*, 152

Bundled payments, 119, 182

Call-coverage issues: comanagement agreements and, 188

Candidates: sourcing, 31

Capital resources: physician acquisitions and, *86*

Capitated (full risk) reimbursement, 155

Capitation, 177

Care coordination: developing/expanding, in Value phase, 160; quality and, in Value phase, 158; shared vision and, 32

Care management: compensation plan redesign and, 155; developing/expanding, in Value phase, 160

Care model: selecting, Value phase and, 17

Care processes: improving, 45. *See also* Quality

Carey, Harry, Jr., 63

Case studies: compensation planning for a tertiary hospital, 125–26; Geisinger Health System, 25; Halifax Health, 22–24; health system in Kentucky, 163–66; health system in the Northeast, 121–24; hospital in the Southeast, 41–42, 99; hospital system in northeast Ohio, 145–47; hospital system in the mid-Atlantic region, 193–95; six-hospital system in the Midwest, 97–98; St. Claire Regional, Kentucky, 38–41; St. Luke's Hospital, Missouri, 143–45; TJ Samson Community Hospital, Kentucky, 77–78

CBO. *See* Central billing office

Centers for Medicare & Medicaid Services (CMS), 162, 208; Transforming Practice Initiative, 156

Central billing office (CBO): for Apex Medical Group, 123, 124; developing and evaluating, 112; establishing, for health system in Northeast, 122; in Operational Chaos phase, 106, *107*. *See also* Billing

CINs. *See* Clinically integrated networks

Clinical and operational emphases: balancing, in High-Performing phase, 171

Clinical integrated networks (CINs): developing or participating, in Value phase, 161–62; fulfilling legal requirements for, 162

Clinical leadership: installing, during Operational Chaos phase, 106, 107, 108

Clinically integrated networks (CINs), 7, 186; designing, 184–85; High-Performing phase and, 176;

management services organizations and, 192; super, 176

Clinical practice: transforming, in Value phase, 156–58

Clinical transformation plan: for employed physician networks, 225

Clinician and Group Consumer Assessment of Healthcare Providers and Systems (CG-CAHPS) metrics, 199

CMS. *See* Centers for Medicare & Medicaid Services

Comanagement agreements, 187–88; base-fee duties in, 187–88; call-coverage issues and, 188; checklist for, *189*; incentive fees and, 187, 188; metric and target selection and, 188; in two-hospital system in mid-Atlantic region case study, 194, 195

Community health: employed networks and, 7

Compensation: aligning with productivity levels, in Operational Chaos phase, 117, *118*; educating physicians about, in Operational Chaos phase, 117, 119, 120; evaluating structure of, 139; operational consistency in Operational Chaos phase and, 110; productivity, 55; staff, 48. *See also* Aligned compensation; Physician compensation

Compensation methodologies: standardizing/optimizing, during Operational Chaos phase, 116–17, *118*, 119

Compensation plans: adopting new, in Value phase, 153–55; redesigning, in Strategic Focus phase, 139–42; redesigning, involving PAC in, 155; simplicity of, 155; for a tertiary hospital (case), 125–26

Competitors: shift to Rapid Growth phase and, 79–80

Compliance documentation: professional services agreements and, 190

Comprehensive Care for Joint Replacement model, 173

Coordination of care: in Value phase, 151

Coppola, Francis Ford, 101

Credentialing: 100-day onboarding plan, in Rapid Growth phase and, 94, 95

Cultural barriers: employed physician networks and, 8

Cultural shift: in Rapid Growth phase, 82

Culture: definition of, 44; in High-Performing employed networks, 44–45; in High-Performing phase, 52, *58*, 169; in HSG Physician Network Evaluation Survey, 229; maintaining, in High-Performing phase, 170–71, 177; in Novice phase, 52, *58*, 66; in Operational Chaos phase, 52, *58*, 104; physician acquisitions and, *86*; in Rapid Growth phase, 52, *58*, 83; in Strategic Focus phase, 52, *58*, 129, *130*; in Value phase, 52, *58*, 151

Customer service measures, 154

Dashboards: areas of focus for, 198–200; central billing office and, 112; definition of, 197; executive-level *vs.* practice management-level information in, 200–201; key purposes of, 197; as a network management tool, 197–219; for Novice networks, 70; sample, 9. *See also* Executive dashboards; Operational dashboards

Data, 50; quality measurement and improvement and, 45; referral management strategy and, 138

Data analytics: lack of infrastructure for, 36; new, integrating in High-Performing phase, 175–76, 177

Data reviews, 20

Deal making: developing consistency in, in Rapid Growth phase, 89–90, 96; establishing standards for, 89

Rapid Growth phase, 94; culture emphasized during, 171; physicians during Rapid Growth phase, 92–95; taking seriously, in Rapid Growth phase, 96; vision and, 33–34

100-day onboarding plan: for every provider, in Rapid Growth phase, 94–95

Operating assessment process: standardized, in Rapid Growth phase, 89–90

Operational Chaos networks: core characteristics of, 103

Operational Chaos phase, 27, 50, 81, 87, 90, 101–26, 131, 136, 201; achieving sustainability goal in, 105; aligned compensation in, 55, 59, 104; brand in, 55, 56, 59, 104; cases, 121–26; culture in, 52, 58, 104; dangers of, 102–3; dashboard metrics for, 208; eight elements in, 103–5; of employed network evolution, 14, 15, 16; financial sustainability in, 50, 56, 59, 105; on growth curve, 102; healthcare organization–based infrastructure in, 101; management infrastructure in, 54, 59, 104; metrics for, 212–13; network evolution from Rapid Growth phase to, 103; "nothing will change" promise made to physicians and, 36; physician leadership in, 53, 58, 104; physician practices in, 101–2; quality in, 52, 53, 58; Rapid Growth phase transition to, reasons for, 81–83; revenue cycle metrics and, 199; sample organizational chart for network moving through, 106, 107; strategy in, 51, 58; value of employed physician network in, 222

Operational Chaos phase, key areas of management focus in, 105–20; engaging providers in network

operations and performance, 112–16; formalizing revenue cycle process, 111–12; installing the right administrative and clinical leaders, 107–10; managing relationship with organizational stakeholders, 119–20; reorganizing and rightsizing the management infrastructure, 105–7; standardizing and optimizing compensation methodologies, 116–17, 119; standardizing and streamlining operational performance, 110–11

Operational dashboards, 198; level of information in, 200–201; sample of, 202–5

Operational efficiency measures, 154

Operationally chaotic networks: characteristics of, 111

Operational performance: standardizing/streamlining during Operational Chaos phase, 110–11

Operations metrics: in dashboards, 200; for evolving networks, 204; for High-Performing phase, 218–19; for Novice phase, 206–7; for Operational Chaos phase, 212–213; for Rapid Growth phase, 210–11; for Strategic Focus phase, 214–215; for Value phase, 216–217

Opioid addiction: battling at St. Claire Healthcare, Kentucky, 163–66

Organizational chart: for network moving through Operational Chaos phase, 106, 107; reinforcing, during Rapid Growth phase, 91

Organizational culture: maintaining, in High-Performing phase, 170–71

Organizational reporting structure: ambiguous, 31

Organizational strategy: aligning with network strategy, 44

Organizational structure: putting in place, in Operational Chaos phase, 106

Professional services agreements (PSAs), 188–91

Profits: risk contracting and, 50

Provider groups: involving same personnel in deal making with, 73

Provider production: operational consistency in Operational Chaos phase and, 110

Providers: educating, in Novice phase, 75; engaging in network's performance, during Operational Chaos phase, 112–16, 120; mix of, broadening under a value-based environment, 172–73, 177; retention of, physician engagement and, 9; strategically targeting, in Rapid Growth phase, 88, 95

PSAs. *See* Professional services agreements

Quadruple Aim: clinically integrated networks and, 184

Quality: definition of, 45; employed physician networks and, 5, 7; in High-Performing employed networks, 45–46; in High-Performing phase, 53, *58*, 169; in HSG Physician Network Evaluation Survey, 233–35; in Novice phase, 52, *58*, 66; in Operational Chaos phase, 52, 53, *58*, 104; physician alignment and, 182; in Rapid Growth Phase, 52, 53, *58*, 83; in Strategic Focus phase, 53, *58*, 129; in Value phase, 53, *58*, 151

Quality-based payment programs: phasing in, 141

Quality improvement: decentralized, 48

Quality metrics, 153, 208; in dashboards, 198–99; for evolving networks, *204*; for High-Performing phase, *218*; for Novice phase, *206*; for Operational Chaos phase, *212*; for Rapid Growth phase, *210*; in

sample operational dashboard, *202*; strategic compensation plan and, 140–41; for Strategic Focus phase, *214*; for Value phase, *216*

Rapid Growth networks: core characteristics of, 80–81

Rapid Growth phase, 50, 75, 79–99; aligned compensation in, 55, *59*, 84; billing in, 111; brand in, 55, *59*, 84; cases, 96–99; culture in, 52, *58*, 83; dashboard metrics of, 208, *210–11*; eight elements in, 83–85; of employed network evolution, *14*, 15, 17; events tied to movement out of, 81; financial sustainability in, *59*, 85; on the growth curve, *80*; issues leading to operational dysfunction in, 82–83; management infrastructure in, 54, *59*, 84; Novice networks entering, factors pushing them into, 65–66; physician leadership in, 53, *58*, 84; quality in, 52, 53, *58*, 83; shift to, reasons for, 79–80; strategy in, 51, *58*, 83; tax IDs in, 106; transition into Operational Chaos phase, reasons for, 81–83; value of employed physician network in, 222

Rapid Growth phase, key areas of management focus in, 87–95; balancing infrastructure development with growth goals, 90–92; controlling the message in medical community, 90; developing consistency in deal making or negotiation, 89–90; executing proactive growth strategy, 87–88; recruiting, acquiring, and onboarding physicians effectively, 92–95

Reactive employment strategy: in Novice phase, 66

Readmission rates, 182

Recruiters: professional, 31

TJ Samson Community Hospital
  (Glasgow, Kentucky) case study,
  77–78
Top-decile performance: achieving, in
  High-Performing phase, 174–75
Triple Aim: clinically integrated networks and, 184
Turnover: provider, proactively
  addressing, 170–71
Two-hospital system in mid-Atlantic
  region (case study), 193–95;
  approach in, 193–94; results in,
  194–95

US Federal Trade Commission, 184
Utilization: physician alignment and,
  182

Value-based care: increased focus on,
  3; strong primary care base and,
  172–73
Value-based purchasing, 119
Value-based reimbursement, 153, 159
Value phase, 50, 129, 149–66, 168;
  aligned compensation in, 55, 59;
  brand in, 56, 59; case, 163–66; culture in, 52, 58; dashboard metrics
  for, 208; eight elements in, 150–52;
  of employed network evolution,
  14, 16, 17; financial sustainability
  in, 56, 59, 152; on growth curve,
  150; management infrastructure
  in, 54, 59; metrics for, 216–17;
  physician leadership in, 54, 58, 151;
  quality in, 53, 58; strategy in, 51–52,
  58; transition from Strategic Focus
  phase to, 150; value of employed
  physician network in, 222
Value phase, key areas of management focus in, 152–62; adopting
  a new compensation plan, 153–55;

developing/expanding care management, care coordination, and
  patient navigation, 160; developing or participating in a clinical integrated network, 161–62;
  improving referral management,
  158; initiating population health
  management program, 160–61,
  162; leveraging the network
  brand in the market, 158–59, 163;
  mobilizing the Physician Advisory
  Council, 152–53; transforming
  clinical practice, 156–58, 162
Value phase network: core characteristics of, 149–50
Vision: development process, 33–34;
  discussions, time frame for, 10; of
  employed physician network, 223
Vision document: drafting, 132
Vision statement: clear, 45
Volume: generating, 7
Volume and throughput metrics: in
  dashboards, 199; for evolving networks, 205; for High-Performing
  phase, 219; for Novice phase, 207;
  for Operational Chaos phase, 213;
  for Rapid Growth phase, 211; in
  sample operational dashboard, 203;
  for Strategic Focus phase, 215; for
  Value phase, 217

Welch, Jack, 221
Workflows: appropriate, central billing
  office and, 112
Work–life balance: younger physicians
  and, 65–66
Work relative value units (wRVUs), 48,
  140, 141; aligning compensation
  with, in Operational Chaos phase,
  117, 118; executive dashboards and,
  199

About the Authors

David W. Miller, FACHE, is managing partner at HSG. His primary areas of focus are strategy development, including strategic plans for hospitals, health systems, and employed physician groups; affiliation/merger strategies; physician alignment strategies; primary care strategies; and service line planning. He also provides board and medical staff education and retreat facilitation.

Before cofounding HSG in 1999, Dave spent four years as a partner at Galvagni-Miller Strategy Group and 15 years as an executive at Norton Healthcare. He is a Fellow of the American College of Healthcare Executives. He holds a master in health administration degree from The Ohio State University and a bachelor in management degree from Virginia Tech.

Terrence R. McWilliams, MD, MSJ, FAAFP, is the chief clinical consultant at HSG. Before joining HSG's consulting team, he spent a decade as the vice president of medical affairs and chief medical officer (CMO) at Newport Hospital. During his tenure as CMO, he supervised the medical staff services office and was responsible for quality of care/patient safety/risk management, clinical information systems, medical staff services, physician recruitment, and clinical service line development. He was intimately involved in numerous systemwide initiatives, including creating the medical staff bylaws, spearheading various clinical information technology projects, and contributing to broad-based performance improvement efforts.

A University of Pittsburgh School of Medicine graduate, Dr. McWilliams retired from the US Navy after a 20-year career as a family physician and clinical administrator in a variety of practice environments, where he led a multispecialty clinical operation and a physician–hospital alignment. He earned a master of science in jurisprudence degree, with a focus on hospital and health law, from Seton Hall University School of Law.

Travis C. Ansel is partner at HSG. In more than ten years as a management consultant, he has worked with a variety of clients, including multihospital tertiary systems and critical access hospitals. His area of focus is helping health systems create structured plans for evolving their physician networks, allowing them to leverage relationships with providers to ensure the system's strategic objectives are being achieved. He believes that physician networks play a crucial role in executing health system strategy and that, to be successful, health system management teams must evolve beyond solely tackling day-to-day decisions and into developing a focused long-term plan for physician network alignment, growth, and capability.

Travis has developed a strong track record of generating revenue growth and growing market share for clients across the country. He partners with each client to understand their landscape and challenges as well as works with management teams and providers to create proactive, implementable plans that will generate success. He brings the right resources to the client to ensure implementation is successful and results are achieved.

He holds a master in business administration degree from Vanderbilt University and dual bachelor of science degrees in finance and business management from the University of Tennessee at Knoxville.